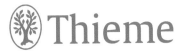

Patient-Centered Communication

The Seven Keys to Connecting with Patients

Natacha J. Moreno, MS, CCC-SLP
Speech-Language Pathologist
Private Practice
Moreno SLP
Largo, Florida

29 illustrations

Thieme
New York • Stuttgart • Delhi • Rio de Janeiro

Library of Congress Cataloging-in-Publication Data

Names: Moreno, Natacha J., author.
Title: Patient-centered communication : the seven keys to connecting with patients / Natacha J. Moreno.
Description: New York : Thieme, [2020] | Includes bibliographical references and index.
Identifiers: LCCN 2019053424 (print) | LCCN 2019053425 (ebook) | ISBN 9781684201839 (paperback) | ISBN 9781684201846 (ebook)
Subjects: MESH: Physician-Patient Relations | Communication | Patient-Centered Care
Classification: LCC R727.3 (print) | LCC R727.3 (ebook) | NLM W 62 | DDC 610.69/6–dc23
LC record available at https://lccn.loc.gov/2019053424
LC ebook record available at https://lccn.loc.gov/2019053425

Important note: Medicine is an ever-changing science undergoing continual development. Research and clinical experience are continually expanding our knowledge, in particular our knowledge of proper treatment and drug therapy. Insofar as this book mentions any dosage or application, readersmay rest assured that the authors, editors, and publishers have made every effort to ensure that such references are in accordance with **the state of knowledge at the time of production of the book.**

Nevertheless, this does not involve, imply, or express any guarantee or responsibility on the part of the publishers in respect to any dosage instructions and forms of applications stated in the book. **Every user is requested to examine carefully** the manufacturers' leaflets accompanying each drug and to check, if necessary in consultation with a physician or specialist, whether the dosage schedules mentioned therein or the contraindications stated by the manufacturers differ from the statements made in the present book. Such examination is particularly important with drugs that are either rarely used or have been newly released on the market. Every dosage schedule or every form of application used is entirely at the user's ownrisk and responsibility. The authors and publishers request every user to report to the publishers any discrepancies or inaccuracies noticed. If errors in this work are found after publication, errata will be posted at www.thieme.com on the product description page.

Some of the product names, patents, and registered designs referred to in this book are in fact registered trademarks or proprietary names even though specific reference to this fact is not always made in the text. Therefore, the appearance of a name without designation as proprietary is not to be construed as a representation by the publisher that it is in the public domain.

Thieme Publishers New York
333 Seventh Avenue, New York, NY 10001 USA
+1 800 782 3488, customerservice@thieme.com

Georg Thieme Verlag KG
Rüdigerstrasse 14, 70469 Stuttgart, Germany
+49 [0]711 8931 421, customerservice@thieme.de

Thieme Publishers Delhi
A-12, Second Floor, Sector-2, Noida-201301
Uttar Pradesh, India
+91 120 45 566 00, customerservice@thieme.in

Thieme Publishers Rio de Janeiro,
Thieme Publicações Ltda.
Edifício Rodolpho de Paoli, 25º andar
Av. Nilo Peçanha, 50 – Sala 2508
Rio de Janeiro 20020-906 Brasil
+55 21 3172 2297

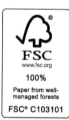

FSC
www.fsc.org
100%
Paper from well-managed forests
FSC® C103101

Cover design: Thieme Publishing Group
Typesetting by Thomson Digital, India

Printed in USA by King Printing Company, Inc.   5 4 3 2 1

ISBN 978-1-68-420183-9

Also available as an e-book:
eISBN 978-1-68-420184-6

To Humberto, Jonathan, and Mackenzie– you all are my everything.

Natacha J. Moreno, MS, CCC-SLP

Contents

Contents

Contents

Videos

Video 1.1 Using positive body language during patient-provider communication

Video 1.2 Using an empathic vocal tone with patients

Foreword

Patient-Centered Communication: The Seven Keys to Connecting with Patients addresses an extremely important topic that lies at the heart of excellence in medical practice–deeply caring communication between caregivers and the individuals they serve.

Society is witnessing the glaring need for compassion and human bonding. Loneliness and social isolationism are reaching shockingly high levels. Healthcare professionals are at the front line of working with people afflicted with both physical and psychological pain. Human bonding is often weak and as a result people experience feelings such as loss, frustration and grief–real or anticipated.

The key task for the caregiver involves building a relationship with the patient by forming an emotional connection. Creating a bond enables caregivers to defuse conflict and de-escalate anxiety, even in the most devastating of circumstances. A trusting and safe environment is essential for the purpose of ensuring psychological safety. The caregiver then becomes a secure base, protecting the patient from all the negative consequences of uncertainty. Caregivers can use meaningful dialogue–talking and listening–to create trust and a positive mindset in order to diffuse fear.

The caregiver's effect, his or her unique impact, be it positive or negative, influences people's health, emotional behavior, and mental state. Since countless healthcare professionals encounter high levels of work-related stress, they are susceptible to burnout now more than ever. This can be attributed, in part, to a diminished feeling of purpose and meaning in their work and personal lives. In addition, overexposure to human pain and suffering can be very destructive. For many, the struggle is a direct consequence of poor, apathetic communication that inhibits bonding with patients, negatively impacting all parties involved.

For many years, Natacha J. Moreno has shared her passion with a diverse group of professionals to form connections with their clients through positive communication. As a speech-language pathologist, she brings to this book an extensive background in coaching clients in the areas of theory of mind, nonverbal communication– the "person effect," and meaningful listening and dialogue. She moves beyond the complexity associated with communication in medicine and offers to her readers a content that focuses on the foundations, which support empathetic dialogue between the caregiver and the patient.

The book shares insights from frontline healthcare professionals across a variety of medical settings and serves as a vital teaching resource. It presents an integrated approach to communication in healthcare by drawing upon the perspectives of multiple disciplines, including hostage negotiation, crisis communication, positive psychology, and social psychology. Highlighted are the critical elements of a healthcare professional's emotional state and the personal effect. It explores how these components directly influence the empathic quality of verbal and, as importantly, nonverbal communication, and their power to bring comfort and lend a new mindset to those in need of healing.

The book engages its readers not only on an intellectual level but also on an emotional one, from evocative real-life patient stories to the heartfelt quotes that introduce each chapter.

For learning to truly take place, however, the reader must be motivated and the target skills practiced. Distinctive features of the book, *Take Action* and *Imagine This*, present opportunities for both. *Imagine This* exercises serve to influence, move, and inspire the reader to act with compassion, while *Take Action* introduces occasions to apply communication skills every day, everywhere, and with everyone.

This book offers a humanistic approach to communication by reinforcing that healing occurs not only in the body but also in the heart and mind. It makes a plea to those who have chosen to serve patients to communicate with compassion and deepen their connection with them.

This is a must read for everyone in the healthcare field and also for those involved in any form of caregiving. Natacha J. Moreno has written an inspiring book!

George Kohlrieser, PhD
Professor
Leadership and Organizational Behavior
International Institute for Management
Development (IMD)
Lausanne, Switzerland

Acknowledgment

This book's creation would not have been possible without the love and support of many. I feel a sense of tremendous gratitude toward my faith that lifts me up and my fellow Marian Servants who exemplify compassion. I would like to thank my colleagues and clients at Lampert's Therapy Group for challenging me to pen this book each and every day. Above all, I am grateful to my husband and children who have proved to be a source of constant encouragement through this remarkable writing journey.

Natacha J. Moreno, MS, CCC-SLP

The Fruits of Compassionate Communication

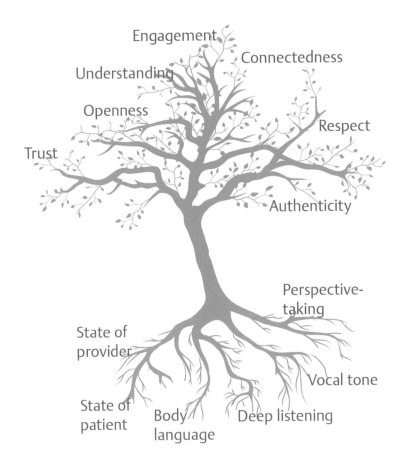

You can't change the fruit without changing the root.
Stephen Covey

The Seven Keys to Compassionate Communication in Health Care

Only the development of compassion and understanding for others can bring us the tranquility and happiness we all seek.

Dalai Lama

Introduction

I had the good fortune of beginning my career in speech-language pathology with an internship at a local children's hospital. The setting offers a wide variety of cases and I was excited about the many learning opportunities awaiting me. What I wasn't quite prepared for were the emotional aspects that accompany working in a medical setting. I was in my early 20s, and had little prior experience of hospitals or of the oftentimes terrifying stories taking place in them. Shy and lacking in confidence, I was afraid I would say the wrong thing, in the wrong way, to patients and parents visibly entrenched in their own fears.

One of my jobs as an intern was to prepare the different consistencies of barium to be used for swallow studies, and then to observe the study, review the outcomes with my mentor, and finally discuss the results and recommendations with the caretaker. One morning, after preparing the barium solutions, our first patient was rolled into the chilly gray suite. Lying on the stretcher was a teenaged girl, quiet and still, with limbs contracted and contorted.

Before the physician arrived, the staff stood in an uneasy silence, staring at this girl—someone's daughter—so alone, so vulnerable to life, and to us. Being a student intern, I wasn't sure of my place, but I remember growing more and more uncomfortable just standing there. Soon, I found myself walking over to her and gently placing my hand on her forearm. Gazing upon her, without uttering a word, I thought "I am with you." With my hand still resting on her arm, my spirit yearned that in some way I was bringing her comfort.

I have no way of knowing how much my touch meant to her, but I know the enduring influence it has had on me. The simple gesture of compassion I was compelled to show another human being is a sweet remembrance that renews me to this day.

It turns out that the way we communicate, both verbally and nonverbally, impacts not only the welfare of the patient, but also our own well-being. There is a reciprocal influence. Neuroscience has demonstrated that communicating with compassion has a myriad of positive effects ranging from decreases in blood pressure, heart rate, and stress hormones to boosts in frontal lobe executive controls that impact creativity, productivity, and decision-making.[1] By the same token, research and testimonies of nurses and physicians suggest that the kindness shown to patients plays as big a role in a patient's healing as the medicines and procedures they undergo.[2]

There is no software program, checklist, in-service, nor handbook in the world that can make providers connect with their clients and patients through the warmth of compassion. While many (including this one) may be important tools for learning, they cannot guarantee that the acquired knowledge is put into action. On the contrary, the intention to communicate with empathy has to originate from within. It must be a conscious, daily, choice to relate to those in our care with patience, humility, vulnerability, and courage. It is, in fact, this opening of our hearts that fills the prescription for compassionate care and delivers a healthy dose of harmony to our work and to our lives.

Getting Started

The book, *Patient-Centered Communication: The Seven Keys to Connecting with Patients*, explores seven critical keys to promoting positive communication that demonstrate compassion toward our clients and patients. They include the following:

- Being mindful of personal state.
- Attending to the patient's emotional state.
- Addressing the patient with the intention to bond.
- Considering the patient's perspective.
- Employing positive body language.
- Listening with the heart and the mind.
- Using vocal tone that reflects empathy.

These keys may also be regarded as the roots or foundation for kind and caring interactions. Once the roots are firmly established, the caregiver and patient can then experience the fruits of compassionate communication.

Each time you pick up the book, prepare yourself mentally and emotionally before beginning to read. This will ensure that you are in the proper state to receive and assimilate the information that is meant to influence your mind and, more importantly, your heart. Take a moment to calm yourself by first becoming conscious of your breath. Continue to relax your body and quiet your thoughts. Adopt the mindset that by engaging with the material in this book you can acquire compassionate communication skills that not only benefit your patients but also bring you a measure of comfort and peace.

Chapter Features

True Patient–Caregiver Stories

Each chapter begins with real-life accounts of communication exchanges between a patient/patient's family member and health care personnel, followed by descriptions of skills associated with the specific key.

When reading the accounts that introduce each section, attempt to adopt the different perspectives of each individual within the story. Imagine yourself as the provider, the patient, or the caretaker—and the impact of the communicative exchange on each person's experience. Look into your heart and remind yourself, "I, too, know what it is like to feel fear, anxiety, anger, and sadness."

Imagine This

Pay attention to the thought bubbles that appear throughout the chapters titled *Imagine This*. These exercises are especially beneficial as empathy stems in part from the ability to imagine what someone else is going through. The feature casts the reader into different everyday situations that promote perspective taking. Not only will *Imagine This* stimulate thinking but it will also potentially inspire the reader to use the highlighted compassionate communication skills with his or her own clients or patients.

Take Action

Each chapter contains text boxes labeled *Take Action*. This feature invites the reader to apply positive verbal and nonverbal communication skills (specific to the chapter) during everyday interactions that can then be carried over to the health care setting. By completing the *Take Action* tasks, readers may become more conscious of certain communication elements of which they may have been previously unaware, or simply disregarded. Most importantly, *Take Action* affords a vital opportunity to put into practice the communication skills being discussed, as opposed to passively learning about them.

References

[1] Doty JR. The Neuroscience of Compassion [Video]. YouTube. https://m.youtube.com/watch?v=Y6pulMOk6do. Published July 21, 2014. Accessed October 25, 2016

[2] Ofri D. What Doctors Feel: How Emotions Affect the Practice of Medicine. Boston, MA: Beacon Press; 2013

Chapter 1

Being Mindful of Personal State

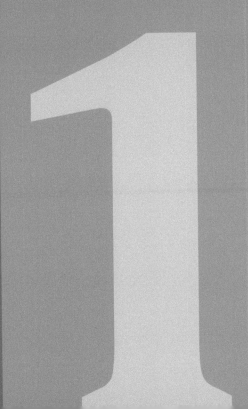

1 Being Mindful of Personal State

Abstract
This chapter explores the significant role of the caregiver's state in determining the quality of patient–provider communication. A provider's state of being is reflected in how he or she approaches and interacts with the patient. It is directly influenced by the body, the mind's eye, personal beliefs, as well as the emotions of others. In the clinical setting, a positive state enables the caregiver to be fully present and engaged in the moment with a patient. Conversely, a negative state can be harmful to the patient's healing process. This chapter introduces the health care professional to a variety of ways to regulate emotions and consequently improve state. Strategies for cultivating mindfulness, nurturing a positive mindset, challenging negative beliefs, and using the mind–body connection to establish presence are outlined. By means of these approaches, the caregiver's resultant positive state can serve as a foundation for successful, patient-centered communication that leads to connection and promotes healing.

Keywords: patient-centered communication, mindfulness, positive mindset, emotional regulation, mind–body connection, patient–provider communication, healing process, mindfulness, establishing presence

Applying focused attention is a moral choice, not just a skill. We pay attention to that which we consider important, and by virtue of paying attention to something, we make it important.

Ronald Epstein, MD

1.1 Taylor's Story

I had been waiting all day for the doctor to drop by mom's room. I decided to postpone going to lunch, and it was a good thing too, because soon there was a knock on the door.

I will refer to the doctor by his first name, Ezra, because I can't recall his last name. I will tell you, though, I remember everything else about him. He was special. The moment he walked through the door, there was a calm confidence about him. He introduced himself, shook my mom's hand, and immediately took a seat. While watching him relax back in his chair, I recall this feeling of relief that overcame me, realizing that this doctor was going to have time for us. Dr. Ezra spoke in an easy way, with a gentle tone and unrushed words. One of the first things he said to my mom was how much he liked her accent and inquired where she was from. It was good to see mom smile and engaged for the first time since she had arrived in the hospital. After a little small talk about mom's hometown, the doctor began to discuss her condition, and the available options for managing her pain. Dr. Ezra even shared a little about his past struggles with back pain. Amazingly, the two bonded in just a short period of time. She told me he had a striking way of making her feel like she had his full attention.

1.2 About State

Regarded as the most important element of communication, an individual's state dictates the success of the communicative exchange. In the medical setting, a caregiver's positive state contributes to being fully present and engaged in the moment with a patient, while a negative state can be detrimental to the healing process.

State is how we are at any specific moment in time and has a direct impact on the quality of our communication with patients. Shaped by the mind's eye, personal beliefs, other's emotions, and the body, our state of being is reflected in how we present ourselves. It encompasses the way we enter a room, how we introduce ourselves, and the manner in which we look and speak to our patients (▶ Fig. 1.1).

Factors relating to the caregiver's level of satisfaction in the workplace can notably influence state as well. For example, the amount of job-related stress they are exposed to and the degree to which they feel valued and supported play a significant role.[1]

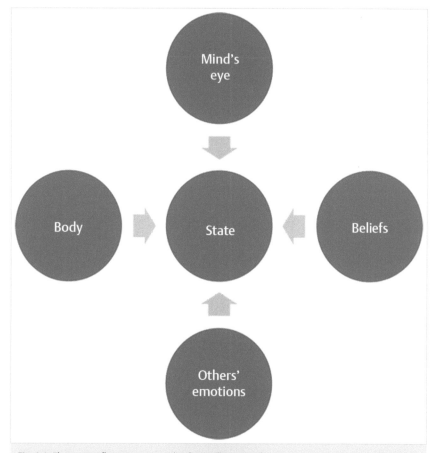

Fig. 1.1 Elements influencing state. This figure illustrates the components impacting the health care professional's disposition during patient interactions.

The caregiver's sense of well-being is also contingent on whether he or she participates in restorative activities. Some activities that are recommended for health care professionals include journaling, meditation, mindfulness exercises, support groups, and wellness training.[2]

1.3 Elements Influencing State

1.3.1 The Mind's Eye

The mind's eye represents a human's ability to visualize things with the mind. It is considered a system of both selective attention and interpretation.[3] Therefore, whatever is in the caregiver's mind's eye will impact how they perceive different aspects of their work and what they choose to focus on—each influencing their state and the way they interact with their patients.

The focus of the mind's eye can allow us to be in the moment with our patients, with thoughts centered around competent, compassionate care. Conversely, when our concentration is on time constraints, quotas, paperwork, office drama, dissenting personnel, difficult bosses, family concerns, etc., it can become an obstacle to presence and engagement. While our focus is elsewhere, we risk suffering from inattentional blindness, or the inability to fully perceive the human being before us. Quieting the mind through contemplative practices like meditation, reflection, and awareness is therefore key. Through continued practice, individuals can begin to view their mental states as something they can control rather than the other way around.[4]

In the midst of life's joys and sorrows, we can choose where we place our attention when we are at work or in the company of a patient. Shawn Achor, an author and expert in the science of happiness and performance, suggests training our brains to constantly pick up on the positives in every situation—what he refers to as the Positive Tetris Effect.[5] In the work setting, for example, we can alter our internal dialogue by overriding the natural human tendency to focus on the negatives of a situation, and instead challenge ourselves with questions that emphasize the potential benefits or pleasures of the job, like the following:

- What is good about my job?
- What is the value of bonding with patients?
- When have clients inspired me?
- How does it benefit me to be fully present and engaged?

By shifting our focus to positive thoughts, we can modify our external perceptions and subsequently improve our ability to connect with our patients.

> **Imagine This #1**
>
> Imagine someone you admire because of his or her ability to always "look on the bright side of things" in spite of personal difficulties. How is this positive mindset reflected in the person's actions? How is it revealed in the words the individual uses to describe their circumstances?

Think of a situation in your life that may be burdensome but may also have a positive side.

1.3.2 Beliefs

Research has shown that the mental construction of our daily activities defines our reality even more than the activity itself.[6] Thus, the beliefs surrounding your job directly impact your state. Positive beliefs inherently result in a favorable state that promote open and empathic communication. Conversely, when the beliefs are negative, not only is work performance compromised, but also the caregiver's verbal and nonverbal behaviors will lack kindness and warmth. To assess your viewpoints, reflect on the following questions: Do I see my job as a chore? Am I just working for a paycheck? Do I feel my position is less important than that of the others? Do I think I am underpaid or unappreciated?

Beliefs can also be in the form of judgments made about patients. For example, do you believe patients are inherently difficult, or even litigious? Have you designated some as unworthy of receiving care? Do you believe certain patients lie or purposely withhold information to achieve their means? The answers to these questions may negatively affect how you approach your interactions with patients, as well as how you interpret them.

Similar to altering the focus of the mind's eye, you can choose to adjust your state by embracing alternative beliefs that will bring meaning to your work and promote feelings of calm and compassion. You can assert:

- It is my calling to serve others in need.
- I am working for this client.
- I am contributing to a greater good.
- The way I approach my patients is integral to their healing.
- Being kind helps the client, and it also helps me.
- All patients deserve care, simply because they are humans.

Imagine This #2 i

Recall an instance when you witnessed an individual being kind and caring to someone you love during a time of need. Recollect the gratitude and perhaps even the relief you felt in your heart. Imagine the unlimited potential of your compassion as you serve your patients.

Another means of adjusting your state is by adopting an optimistic explanatory style or a positive way of interpreting adversity.[5] For example, you can elect to favorably frame situations like the following:

- The patient is behaving poorly toward me because he is fearful and suffering.
- This challenge is giving me an opportunity to shine.
- I do not get the recognition I feel I deserve because my boss is overwhelmed.
- I did not get a raise, but this job allows me to pay my bills.
- All I can do is my very best.

1.3.3 Other People's Emotions

Just as a caregiver's state can affect the patient, the reverse is also true. In fact, our state is highly susceptible to the emotionally charged patients and situations we encounter.

Witnessing the raw, painful emotions of a patient has the power to influence how we feel because emotions can be contagious. Daniel Goleman, author of *Social Intelligence*, affirms that, "Like secondhand smoke, the leakage of emotions can make a bystander an innocent casualty of someone else's toxic state."[7] This occurs because emotions spread from person to person as a result of two aspects of human interaction. We are biologically hardwired to mimic others and in mimicking their outward displays, we adopt their inward states.[8]

Take Action #1

Choose an emotion among the following: anger, sadness, fear, disgust, surprise, and happiness. Find an image of a person displaying that emotion intensely on the internet. After looking at the picture for a few moments, note the changes in the way your face and body feel. Did you begin to feel the emotion as well?

In the midst of the patient's struggle, the caregiver's objective is to be mindful of observing, understanding, and regulating his or her own emotional reactions in order to maintain presence.[4] Like other variables affecting state, counteracting another person's adverse state must be a conscious choice and is contingent upon accepting that you are not at the mercy of your emotions.[9] Employing the neocortex ("thinking" brain), you can override the emotions from the reptilian brain and the limbic system and avert becoming hostage to automatic emotional reactions.[3] While challenging, with awareness and practice, you can take control of your emotions instead of your emotions having control over you. To do this, renowned psychologist, Paul Ekman, advises engaging in emotional consciousness, wherein you must first become aware an emotion is surfacing, and then take a step back. Next, as you are experiencing the emotion, you become like a mindful onlooker questioning or considering the best course of action to respond to the emotion.[8] If the situation calls for an empathetic response, a compassionate action will help relieve some of the unavoidable emotional tension you are undergoing.[4]

To thwart painful emotions, also consider keeping a picture of someone you love close at hand. Gazing at the photograph may prompt mimicking of a pleasant facial expression or evoking of positive emotions, with both actions serving to restore composure. Another way to reset uncomfortable emotions is to step away for a few minutes to engage in something pleasurable that is unrelated to work, such as watching a funny video clip, listening to a joyful song, reading a comic strip, etc.

In the cases where a patient has exhibited rude or unkind behavior, it may be helpful to refer to an old thank you card or note from someone who has appreciated you. Reading it will help you shake off any negativity and remind you of your worth.

1.3.4 The Body

By virtue of the profession, health care professionals are habitually under varying degrees of stress. Exposure to suffering, sorrow, and fear can spur cognitive and emotional reactions that result in bodily changes such as muscle tension, rapid, shallow breathing or holding of breath, and facial expressions mimicking the struggling patient (▶ Fig. 1.2).

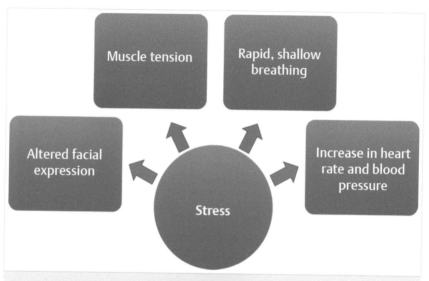

Fig. 1.2 Bodily reactions to stress. Shown are physical effects a caregiver may experience as a result of emotional distress during patient–provider interactions.

For this reason, a major challenge for caregivers is readjusting their state in between difficult patient cases. When this important step is not taken, small stresses pile up that can lead to emotional distress in the form of anger, irritability, and anxiety. Quick strategies are thus needed to de-stress and to reestablish presence.

Take Action #2

Being available and present to your client/patient requires mindful awareness—the ability to sit down quietly and connect with yourself. Take the next few moments to breathe in and out and reflect on what is currently going on in your body, including your perceptions and feelings.

You may also try this exercise "Where are my feet?" to practice establishing a mindful state.[4] For a few moments, concentrate solely and completely on your two feet—noting their position relative to the floor and whether one is supporting more weight than the other. Are there any feelings of aches or pains or other sensations? In times of stress, it is suggested to return to this exercise to regain calm and focus.

Taking deep breaths between visits can be just the remedy for becoming fully present for the next patient. Several deliberate breaths, also known as recovery breaths, will help restore equilibrium and signal to your body that all is well. Deeply inhale through the mouth and watch your belly expand. Then pay special attention to lengthening the exhalation; when done slowly, it triggers the parasympathetic nervous system and slows down the heart rate.[10] Information from the lungs and heart is fed back to the brain and convinces it that things are calm and peaceful even if they are not.[10]

Imagine a professional tennis player getting ready to serve a tennis ball—from the number of times they choose to bounce the ball, to the height at which the ball is bounced and then tossed into the air. Each action is performed intentionally and methodically. This is referred to as a performance preparation routine and is a linchpin for top-notch performers like star athletes and world-class musicians. Through these personalized routines, the individual engages in systematic thoughts and actions prior to the performance activity that regulate arousal and concentration, thus maximizing performance.[11]

What could be your preperformance routine to use before approaching each patient/client that would help you to relax, focus, and prepare mentally to be fully present for them?

As we approach clients and patients, the way we use our bodies plays a major role in determining our state. This is due to the mind–body connection, wherein what we do with the body affects the mind, and vice versa.

Scientific evidence suggests that emotional change can be achieved by altering a physical behavior, such as modifying facial expression and posture.[5] To attain a sense of calm, for example, you can drop your shoulders and consciously relax your chest and throat as you breathe. At the same time, consider smiling regardless of how you feel, as studies have shown that it helps individuals' ability to recover from stressful events.[12] The act of smiling reduces the level of stress-enhancing hormones like cortisol, adrenaline, and dopamine, while increasing the level of mood-enhancing hormones like serotonin.[13] Even if you are forcing a smile, it can end up making you feel happier, as our neural circuitry does not always differentiate between what is fake and what is real.[14]

In her book, *Presence: Bringing Your Boldest Self to Your Biggest Challenges*, social psychologist Amy Cuddy recommends another method of tapping into the mind–body connection to positively affect state. She explains: "Expanding your body physiologically prepares you to be present; it overrides your instinct to fight or flee, allowing you to be grounded, open, and engaged."[15] Through her experiments on expansive postures—such as placing hands on the hips or extending the arms over the head to enlarge the body—it was found that by simply having subjects engage in these poses resulted in feelings of presence and personal power (▶ Fig. 1.3 and ▶ Fig. 1.4).

A large part of our day is spent interfacing with our computers, tablets, and smartphones. As a result, we are sitting for long blocks of time in postures that are likely to be unhealthy or closed. Our torsos may be leaning forward with our necks extended toward a computer screen, or when on a tablet or phone, our shoulders and head may be hunched.

The next time you spend an extended period on one of your devices, take a few moments to stand or perhaps walk around. Adjust the positioning of your body and adopt an expansive posture. Are you able to note any changes in the way you are feeling both mentally and physically?

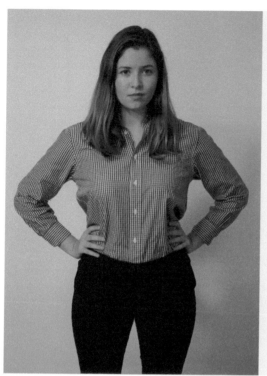

Fig. 1.3 Expansive body posture spurring feelings of presence and personal power.

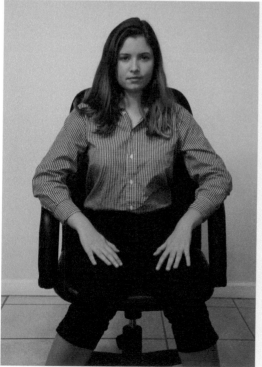

Fig. 1.4 Expansive body posture while sitting.

Summary

Comments from patient focus groups reveal that when caregivers are in an adverse state, these feelings are palpable to patients.[16] To promote wellness in others, health care professionals must work in an environment where they personally feel cared for and valued, as well as invest in their own self-management. Cultivating a positive mindset and challenging negative beliefs, as well as being aware of how others' states affect us, will also assist caregivers in treating patients with mindful engagement. When all of these factors come together, the resulting positive state will serve as a foundation for successful, compassionate communication that leads to connection and promotes healing.

References

[1] Spiegelman P, Berrett B. Patients come second: leading change by changing the way you lead. Austin, TX: Greenleaf Book Group; 2013

[2] Sanchez-Reilly S, Morrison LJ, Carey E, et al. Caring for oneself to care for others: physicians and their self-care. J Support Oncol. 2013; 11(2):75–81

[3] Kohlrieser G. Hostage at the table: how leaders can overcome conflict, influence others, and raise performance. San Francisco, CA: Jossey-Bass; 2006

[4] Epstein R. Attending: medicine, mindfulness, and humanity. New York, NY: Scribner; 2017

[5] Achor S. The happiness advantage: the seven principles that fuel success and performance at work. New York, NY: Crown Publishing Group; 2010

[6] Crum AJ, Langer EJ. Mind-set matters: exercise and the placebo effect. Psychol Sci. 2007; 18(2):165–171

[7] Goleman D. Social intelligence. New York, NY: Bantam; 2006

[8] Ekman P. Emotions revealed: recognizing faces and feelings to improve communication and emotional life. New York, NY: St. Martin's Griffin; 2007

[9] Feldman Barrett L. You aren't at the mercy of your emotions—your brain creates them. [video]. YouTube. https://www.youtube.com/watch?v=0gks6ceq4eQ, Published January 23, 2018. Accessed March 22, 2018

[10] Bell B. MD. How your breath affects your nervous system. https://featheredpipe.com/breath-affects/. Published 2018. Accessed August 24, 2018

[11] Muran A. Emotion regulation and pre-performance routines in competitive sports. Res Investigations Sports Med. 2018; 3(4):1:3

[12] Kraft TL, Pressman SD. Grin and bear it: the influence of manipulated facial expression on the stress response. Psychol Sci. 2012; 23(11):1372–1378

[13] Gutman, R. The hidden power of smiling. PsycEXTRA Dataset. 2011. Available at: https://www.ted.com/talks/ron_gutman_the_hidden_power_of_smiling/transcript?language=en

[14] Beilock S. How the body knows its mind. London: Robinson; 2015

[15] Cuddy AR. Presence: bringing your boldest self to your biggest challenges. New York, NY: Little, Brown and Company; 2015

[16] Frampton S. Patient-centered care: improvement guide. Derby, CT: Planetree; 2008

Chapter 2

Attending to the Patient's State

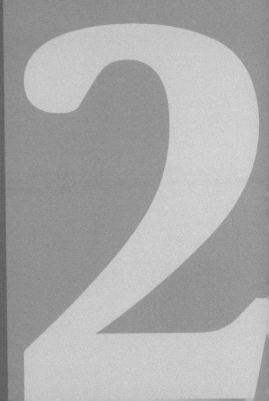

2 Attending to the Patient's State

Abstract

This chapter introduces approaches to facilitate change in the distressed patient's state through a mutual transaction. As patients grapple with negative emotions, their executive functions are compromised. Conversation becomes significantly more taxing. As a result, the quality of the patient–provider communication is adversely affected and the patient's healing process is simultaneously impeded. This chapter outlines specific strategies to assist in moderating a patient's state, including asking questions, minding vocal tone and speech delivery, and feeding information back to the patient. Additionally, visual and auditory indicators are listed for four prevailing emotions in the health care setting (sorrowful, angry, fearful, and defensive), accompanied by verbal and nonverbal communication strategies to defuse each of those states. In moderating the patient's state, cognitive functioning improves, rendering it more conducive to the process and exchange of information.

Keywords: executive functions, cognitive functioning, distressed patients, patients' emotional states, negative emotions, patient–provider communication, healing process, communication strategies

If an individual has a calm state of mind, that person's attitudes and views will be calm and tranquil even in the presence of great agitation.

                                                                    Dalai Lama

2.1 Jenny's Story

I needed to have an MRI done on my brain. Two years had passed since my head injury, and I was still having some lingering symptoms.

The facility I went to was small and clean, but everything seemed so overwhelming and loud to me. Right from the start, I alerted the technician that I had sound sensitivity and anxiety. He said not to worry—he would give me some earplugs and that would help. I was so relieved that he actually listened to me. Normally, when I go in for a scan, the technicians are super busy prepping everything and they don't really even look at me. He was different. He looked at me as though he could really see me.

The MRI machine was huge, and it was housed in a tiny room that barely seemed to fit it. I started to tremble a little, probably because the room was cold, and my nerves kicked in. He got me set up in the machine, complete with a blanket, earplugs, and a masque for my eyes—everything to help me feel grounded. Just before he left the room, he touched my forearm. It was just a brief touch, but enough to communicate that he cared and that I was going to be okay.

I marvel over the profound shift from being overridden with anxiety as I entered the facility, to feeling calm and grounded as I reclined in the MRI. I truly believe the change came from being listened to, cared for, and acknowledged through touch. "I get you, I got you, we're good"—that is what I feel he communicated to me.

2.2 About the Patient's State

Fearful, vulnerable, agitated, and overwhelmed are just some of the words that can describe patients' emotional states. Oftentimes, they find themselves in unfamiliar surroundings, inundated with foreign terms and drowning in new information. In many cases, patients do not know what their clinical status is, nor what the outcome will be, and worry about how their condition might affect their lives.

As patients grapple with a wide range of emotions, it becomes increasingly challenging for them to acclimate to the novel workings of a medical setting. With feelings of powerlessness comes a decline in clear thinking, and they may struggle meeting the demands of their complicated and stressful situation.[1] Executive functions, such as reasoning, planning, attention control, and working memory are all compromised with the rise of negative emotions.[1] In turn, when these cognitive functions are undermined, conversation becomes significantly more taxing for these individuals, as evidenced in slower speech, delayed response times, and more pauses.[2] A clear example of this challenge is described by Jerod Loeb, PhD, former Joint Commission's executive vice president of Healthcare Quality Evaluation. In regard to a frightening personal patient experience, he states "…I become deaf, dumb, and blind. I hear nothing, I listen to nothing. I am unable to repeat what has been just told to me…." (▶ Fig. 2.1)

Imagine This #1

Imagine a time when you experienced a significant emotional reaction (i.e., news of a loss, getting a driving ticket, a public speaking engagement). Was it hard to formulate thoughts in that moment? How difficult was it to find the words you wanted to say? Afterward, did you struggle recalling what was said to you?

Now consider the cognitive strain patients experience when clutched by their emotions.

Even in cases where a caregiver clearly and wholly provides information to the patient, a communication breakdown can occur if the patient is not in the right state to receive it. For this reason, when a patient is exhibiting signs of emotional distress, it is imperative that the caregiver address those feelings first. Leonard Greenberger, author

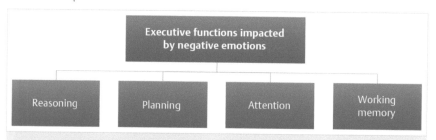

Fig. 2.1 Executive functions impacted by negative emotions. Represented in this figure are the four cognitive processes adversely affected in distressed patients. The subsequent decline in mental functioning directly influences the quality of the patient–provider communication.

of *What to Say When Things Get Tough*, warns: "If we don't address and calm emotions first, the facts, data, and information we try to communicate will (figuratively) bounce off people's emotions." In health care, gaps in the patient's understanding of his diagnosis, condition, and next steps are clear evidence of when state is ignored.

One solution is for caregivers to employ strategies used in the science of hostage negotiation—a profession that routinely transforms individuals' states in high-stakes situations. The psychological principles and practices of hostage negotiations may be applied to the resolution of interpersonal crisis across many domains,[3] including the ones patients routinely encounter in the medical setting.

To that end, George Kohlrieser, clinical psychologist and veteran hostage negotiator, suggests proven techniques that facilitate change in another person's state through a mutual transaction.[4] Specifically, he recommends communication strategies that hostage negotiators employ to lower the hostage taker's state of arousal and that can be used in other stressful situations. Kohlrieser's strategies, outlined in the following sections, have been adapted for the health care professional to assist in moderating a patient's state, rendering it more conducive to processing and exchanging information.

2.3 Moderating a Patient's State

2.3.1 Address the Patient with the Intention to Bond

Approach the patient with the mindset of making him feel heard, cared for, and understood. Use the first critical minutes to establish a bond or an emotional connection that will lead to trust. Engage in open body postures and express energy and warmth.[4]

2.3.2 Maintain a Calm State

Caregivers are called upon to regulate their own emotions while considering the patient's emotional state. Taking deep breaths or squeezing your hands tightly may help ground you in the face of strong emotions.[5] The aim is to present in a calm state that will, in turn, be reflected in a serene tone of voice. This sense of calm will automatically spread to the patient. You can also maintain your composure by engaging in active listening, as the cardiac-orienting reflex will be activated and will lower your physiological state of arousal.[4]

Imagine This #2　　　　　　　　　　　　　　　　　　　　　　　　　　　　　　ⓘ

When you appear relaxed, the person with whom you are interacting can begin to relax as well. Imagine you are in the company of someone with whom you feel calm and comfortable. Identify the pattern in your body, face, and breath that signifies the feeling of being relaxed. How do the muscles in your face feel? Are your shoulders up or down? Is your breathing deep or shallow? Form a memory of this somatic sense of tranquility.

It is important that the caregiver does not appear to be rushed, as this will only exacerbate the patient's distress. When emotions are high, patients need to feel they have the time and space to hear, assimilate, and process the information they are being given.

Take Action #1

After completing **Imagine This 2**, recall and practice the behaviors that signify your relaxed state as you carry out daily routines. Next, practice these same qualities in situations that are more stressful—waiting in line, caught up in traffic, managing bills, etc. With repetition, reverting to a relaxed state will become a response that can be called upon to regulate emotions in difficult situations, such as treating a distressed client or patient.

2.3.3 Ask Questions to Lower State of Arousal

Pose open-ended questions to focus the patient's mind's eye, as well as lower states of arousal, blood pressure, and heart rate.[4] This will assist in regulating listening and will help diffuse the tension of the situation. Additionally, answers provide the caregiver with valuable information regarding the patients' perspective. Some examples of open-ended questions/statements include the following:

- What is worrying you?
- Tell me more.
- Help me to understand.

2.3.4 Pay Attention to Vocal Tone and Speech Delivery

Using a calm voice can itself help reduce the pressure of a situation. By speaking slowly and clearly, you will be modeling how you want the conversation to progress. Next, adapt your conversation level to that of the patient's. Avoid medical jargon and vocabulary that may be "over" his head.

Imagine This #3

Using complex medical terms can cause confusion and diminish understanding between the health care professional and the patient. This in turn leads to feelings of anxiety in the patient and directly impedes trust and confidence.

Imagine a time when someone was explaining something to you of importance and the individual used many words that you did not comprehend. How did it make you feel? Were you in the best state to process all of the information or to make decisions? Consider this when you provide explanations to your patients.

2.3.5 Feed Information Back to Patient

Feeding information back to the patient is a form of acknowledgment and an essential step in building trust. It will allow him to feel heard and simultaneously improve his state.

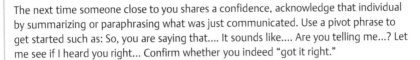

Take Action #2 ✔

The next time someone close to you shares a confidence, acknowledge that individual by summarizing or paraphrasing what was just communicated. Use a pivot phrase to get started such as: So, you are saying that.... It sounds like.... Are you telling me...? Let me see if I heard you right... Confirm whether you indeed "got it right."

2.4 Patients' Emotional States

Perception springs from presence, meaning the health care provider must be focused and engaged to tune into the patient's emotions. Any number of markers can reveal how the patient is feeling, including body postures, gestures, facial expressions, and tone of voice. When caregivers activate all of the senses necessary to decipher these silent and verbal cues, they can discern the patient's emotional state and respond in an empathic way.[6]

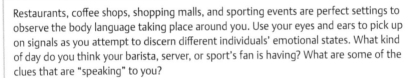

Take Action #3 ✔

Restaurants, coffee shops, shopping malls, and sporting events are perfect settings to observe the body language taking place around you. Use your eyes and ears to pick up on signals as you attempt to discern different individuals' emotional states. What kind of day do you think your barista, server, or sport's fan is having? What are some of the clues that are "speaking" to you?

While patients exhibit a wide variety of emotions, outlined below are a few states that prevail in the health care setting. If the patient's emotional state is indeed compromised, the caregiver can implement effective strategies that will reestablish equilibrium so that they are better able to intake information and to communicate more effectively.

2.4.1 The Sorrowful State

A depiction of the sorrowful state is shown in ▶ Fig. 2.2.

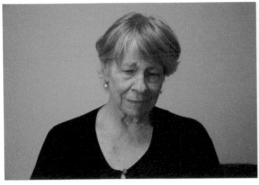

Fig. 2.2 The sorrowful state.

Visual indicators of the sorrowful state are as follows: head down, lowering of gaze, pouted or compressed lips, frowning eyebrows and mouth, and slumping shoulders with upper body downward.[7]

Audible indicators are as follows: higher-than-average pitch; less intensity (loudness); frequent, long pauses; and flat speech tone, when compared with neutral speech.[8]

De-escalating the Sorrowful State

Foremost, the patient's distress must be acknowledged. This can be accomplished in part by labeling the presenting emotion, which will in turn lead the patient to feel validated.

Next, showing concern is essential, as it provides emotional healing to a patient who is deeply saddened. Through the caregiver's empathic response, the patient is able to feel that his pain is seen and that there is genuine regard for his state.

Empathy can be demonstrated both verbally and nonverbally. Nonverbal methods may involve using a soft, lower tone of voice; tilting the head; placing a hand over the heart;[9] touching the patient's hand or shoulder; mirroring the patient's facial expression; and using open body postures and gestures. Verbally, encouraging words and statements can be made, such as: "I am here for you;" "I wish I could ease some of your sadness;" or "I can only imagine how difficult this must be." Also consider pausing after providing an empathic statement to allow the patient the space to share his fears, values, and hopes.[10]

If the empathic response does not arrive naturally to you, try using your imagination to promote understanding by posing questions like: What would I do in this situation? If this happened to me, how would I feel?[11] In that moment of imagination, it may be possible to tune into the emotions your patient may be experiencing.

2.4.2 The Angry State

A depiction of the angry state is shown in ▶ Fig. 2.3.

Visual indicators of the angry state are as follows: clenching jaw, tense mouth, eyebrows down with vertical furrows above the nose, flared nostrils, and clenching hands into tight fists.[7]

Audible indicators include the following: low pitch with higher intensity (raised voice) when compared with neutral speech.[8]

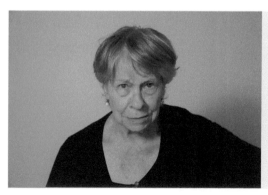

Fig. 2.3 The angry state.

De-escalating the Angry State

Most importantly, be mindful of your own state. Try to remain calm by becoming conscious of your breath and reminding yourself not to take the patient's angry words or actions personally.

The immediate goal is for the patient to regain composure, and this is best accomplished by giving him the conversational floor without interrupting.[12] Allowing the patient to completely vent about the problem is the only way to quiet the irate voice in his mind. During this time, ask clarifying questions that will promote elaboration on what he is going through, and at the same time will signal to him that you have been listening. Finally, paraphrase what you have heard. This will give him additional confirmation that you have listened well and are aware of his viewpoint.

In addition to active listening, connect with him by showing empathy. When the patient feels empathized with, his state of arousal will automatically decrease.[11] Consider using phrases that will help to connect with his feelings, like, "I wouldn't like that either;" or "I would be very angry as well."

In some cases, it may be necessary to issue an apology. Be mindful that how you say something is far more important than what you say. The patient needs to feel you are being authentic, or else you are literally and figuratively wasting your breath.

2.4.3 The Fearful State

A depiction of the fearful state is shown in ► Fig. 2.4.

Visual indicators of the fearful state are as follows: trembling teeth/lips, fast eye blinking, muscle tension, tense or open mouth, sweating,[7] widened eyes, fidgeting, wringing of hands, fingers in mouth, self-soothing gestures,[13] lip licking, puffing out of cheeks, and slowly exhaling.[14]

Audible indicators include the following: vocal tremors, higher pitch with little variation, faster speech rate, and more pauses when compared with neutral speech.[8]

De-escalating the Fearful State

Patients in a fearful state feel powerless, and this feeling can become a major obstacle to healing. As with the other patient states, it is important to ask questions to lower the state of arousal. Provide an opening for the patient to freely discuss his feelings by using simple probes like, "What are your concerns?" or "What is worrying you?" Listen well

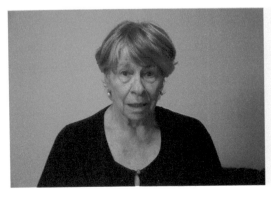

Fig. 2.4 The fearful state.

and provide a compassionate response that validates what the patient is experiencing, like, "It can be scary when...." By the same token, avoid the phrase, "Yes, but...." It discounts whatever was said before and minimizes the individual's concerns.

Knowledge is the patient's gateway to abating fears and rebuilding personal power. Gaining a clearer understanding of the diagnosis, treatment options, stages of recovery, etc., is a necessary step in regaining a sense of control. When communicating with the fearful patient, avoid ambiguity, and opt for direct, honest conversation. Armed with clarity, he will then feel in a better position to ask questions and to be a part of the decision-making process.

2.4.4 The Defensive State

A depiction of the defensive state is shown in ▶ Fig. 2.5.

Visual indicators of the defensive state are as follows: closed-body postures and gestures such as clenched hands, crossed arms, legs, and ankles, hands in the pockets,[13] and pursed lips.[14]

Audible indicators—not specified in literature—may include any combination of angry and fearful vocal markers.

De-escalating the Defensive State

The patient who feels defensive is one who might possess a differing perspective surrounding his illness. He may arrive wanting a certain test, procedure, therapy, or prescription because he feels it is what is best for him, and at the same time, he is afraid of being denied what he wants. In the end, the goal is for the patient to feel understood by the caregiver, as well as comprehend his or her explanations. Joshua Kosowsky, physician and author, speaks about the negotiation that sometimes takes place between him and his patients: "When my patients come in asking for a test or a prescription that I don't think they need, I tell them that I'll make a deal with them: they have to hear me out and I have to hear them out, and at the end, we'll make the decision together."[15]

For productive communication to take place, the caregiver must attend to the patient's guarded state. Like the fearful state, it requires conversing with the patient in a way that engenders trust and credibility. The caregiver must first demonstrate authentic empathy and care. Together, they are the most important criterion by which people judge whether or not one is a trustworthy and credible person and source of information.[16]

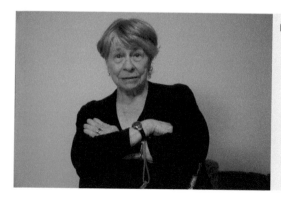

Fig. 2.5 The defensive state.

Following are some key strategies that may render the patient in a less defensive state and promote a more constructive communicative exchange:

- Let the patient talk first and key in on his perspective. Allow him the time and space to voice his concerns and what he feels may help him and why. Use statements like "Help me understand what makes this the best option for you"[9] to find out what is motivating him, and this will in turn help lead the focus of the dialogue.
- Show sincere and authentic interest in what the patient wants. Recognize his feelings and views by making statements such as: "I can see you have strong feelings about this. Help me understand your concerns." In this way, you are not endorsing the patient's opinion, but affirming his right to have a differing point of view. The patient will immediately feel he has been heard and treated with respect and, therefore, is less likely to maintain a defensive stance.
- Mirror the patient's conversational level. Use clear, succinct, straightforward language that will make him more apt to trust you.
- Speak to your patient's concerns and goals and highlight areas of differences and agreement. Explain the reasons behind why you are recommending for something to be done, or not to be done. Sometimes all it takes to calm the defensive patient is to enlighten him of benefits, risks, and side effects.[15]

Summary

While strapped for time, caregivers must resist the temptation to "get right down to business" with patients who are visibly distressed. In those moments, it is important to remind ourselves that healing involves attending to those difficult feelings, and not simply treating the body. Moreover, when we take the time to address feelings first, it helps the patient to regain composure and leads to a more effective communication exchange.

References

[1] Cuddy AR. Presence: bringing your boldest self to your biggest challenges. New York, NY: Little, Brown and Company; 2015

[2] Greene JO, Ravizza SM. Complexity effects on temporal characteristics of speech. Hum Commun Res. 1995; 21(3):390–421

[3] Miller L. Hostage negotiation: psychological principles and practices. Int J Emerg Ment Health. 2005; 7(4): 277–298

[4] Kohlrieser G. Hostage at the table: how leaders can overcome conflict, influence others, and raise performance. San Francisco, CA: Jossey-Bass; 2006

[5] Lampert L. Emotional patients: how to maintain professionalism. https://www.ausmed.com/articles/emotional-patients/ Published 2016. Accessed April 15, 2018

[6] Goleman D. Focus: the hidden driver of excellence. New York, NY: HarperCollins; 2015

[7] Givens DB. The nonverbal dictionary. http://center-for-nonverbal-studies.org/htdocs/6101.html. Accessed July 10, 2018

[8] Sauter DA, Eisner F, Calder AJ, Scott SK. Perceptual cues in nonverbal vocal expressions of emotion. Q J Exp Psychol (Hove). 2010; 63(11):2251–2272

[9] Boissy A, Gilligan T. Communication the Cleveland clinic way: how to drive a relationship-centered strategy for superior patient experience. New York, NY: McGraw-Hill Education; 2016

[10] October TW, Dizon ZB, Arnold RM, Rosenberg AR. Characteristics of physician empathetic statements during pediatric intensive care conferences with family members: a qualitative study. JAMA Netw Open. 2018; 1(3): e180351

[11] Lee F. If Disney ran your hospital: 9 1/2 things you would do differently. Bozeman, MT: Second River Healthcare Press; 2004

[12] Meyers P, Nix S. As We Speak: How to Make Your Point and Have It Stick. New York, NY: Atria Paperback; 2012

[13] Pease A, Pease B. The definitive book of body language. New York, NY: Bantam Books; 2006

[14] Navarro J, Karlins M. What every BODY is saying: an ex-FBI agent's guide to speed-reading people. New York, NY: HarperCollins; 2015

[15] Wen LS, Kosowsky JM. When doctors don't listen: how to avoid misdiagnoses and unnecessary tests. New York, NY: Thomas Dunne Books; 2014

[16] Greenberger LS. What to say when things get tough: business communication strategies for winning people over when they're angry, worried and suspicious of everything ou say. New York, NY: McGraw-Hill Education; 2013

Chapter 3

Considering the Patient's Perspective

3 Considering the Patient's Perspective

Abstract

This chapter offers a myriad of verbal and nonverbal communication skills that can be used to become better attuned to the patient and promote patient-centered communication. It introduces the reader to strategies that will assist in seeing the patient's situation through their eyes—including cultural considerations, the way they view their illness and prognosis, and what they feel is the optimal course of treatment. In addition, it discusses the importance of promoting health literacy to improve adherence of treatment plans. This chapter also examines how perspective-taking requires understanding and accepting that others have beliefs, desires, intentions, and viewpoints that are different from our own. In other words, staff must be able to respect and see the "whole" patient. Through this perspective-taking process, the caregiver can more effectively address the patient's social, emotional, and physical needs, and ultimately improve treatment outcomes.

Keywords: perspective-taking, patient-centered communication, compassionate communication, "whole" patient, health literacy, cultural considerations, adherence of treatment plans

Those who are without compassion cannot see what is seen with the eyes of compassion.
Thich Nhat Hanh

3.1 Madeline's Story

Many years ago, the members of my nursing class interned at a large intercity county hospital where we were assigned to the men's medical ward. There were homeless men, poor men, and even men shackled to their beds—all housed in a large room crammed with 60 beds arranged neatly in rows. It was by no means an easy assignment for us naïve, young interns.

One day, I was caring for a patient when I overheard a fellow intern, Amy, instructing in her characteristically prim and proper tone, "Sir, I need you to give me a urine specimen." She was holding a specimen cup to the patient, and he just sat there with a confused look on his face. She repeated the same request multiple times, each time raising her voice louder and louder as if it would somehow help him to better understand what she was saying. His cheeks began to blush, and he lowered his gaze.

Due to the way the beds were arranged, our supervisor, Ms. Leeann, could see the whole debacle unfolding. She quickly made her way over to Amy, grasped the cup, and in a hushed voice said to the patient, "Piss in the can." The man's face immediately lit up in recognition.

To this day, I enjoy a hearty laugh as I recall the shocked look on Amy's face over Ms. Leeann's blunt speech. More importantly, though, I feel tremendous gratitude for the valuable lesson I learned that day. Through the years of working with patients from all walks of life, I have realized the importance of trying to see things through their eyes—figuring out where they are coming from and speaking to them on their level.

3.2 Perspective-Taking

In the medical setting, the patient's perspective refers to how they view their illness and the social and psychological ramifications surrounding it. Perception may be influenced by cultural, religious, and spiritual beliefs and in turn impacts the way they approach their illness as well as the care they receive. To connect with patients, staff must be able to respect and see the patient as a "whole" individual, as well as take in the broad view of the patient's situation in that moment in time.

> **Imagine This #1**
>
> Consider a financially struggling client who must take a bus or rely on others for transportation to access health care services. Beyond the physical concerns of their condition, what anxieties might the individual be grappling with in terms of getting treatment? How might addressing these worries be therapeutic to the patient? Imagine the positive impact a sympathetic comment could have on the patient–caregiver relationship.

Perspective-taking entails trying to see the patient's circumstances through their eyes. It therefore requires understanding and accepting that others have beliefs, desires, intentions, and viewpoints that are different from our own. In the end, getting the patient's perspective is what enables us to effectively address their social, emotional, and physical needs and to ultimately build their trust. Furthermore, it facilitates patient-centered communication, such as considering the patient's desire for information and joint decision-making.[1]

> **Take Action #1**
>
> Patient-centered communication is key to acquiring the patient's perspective. It entails both careful listening and tactful strategic questioning.
>
>   Use the many opportunities in your daily life to practice these two vital communication skills. Consider a difference of opinion that you have with someone who is close to you. Focus specifically on the words the two of you have exchanged. Come up with three or four questions you could ask the individual to gain a better perspective of their viewpoint.

3.3 Cultural Competence

Caregivers can show respect to their patients by adjusting their mode of interaction accordingly. This involves demonstrating attitudes and behaviors that are sensitive to the values, customs, and ethnic backgrounds of their patients, while keeping in mind that those patients may have a completely different understanding of their illness.[2] Patients from varied cultures may also have alternative explanations for why they are experiencing a specific event, as well as differing priorities when it comes to treatment goals.

In addition to researching the cultural characteristics of target patient populations, it is critical for the caregiver to discuss the patient's beliefs with them, including how they view their prognosis and what they feel is the optimal treatment.[1] When these beliefs are incorporated into the treatment plan, acceptance and compliance of that plan improves.[3]

Imagine This #2

Imagine you are seeking treatment for a condition (i.e., colitis, asthma, sleep apnea, irregular heart beat) and your belief in what is causing the condition completely differs from the one proposed by the health care professional. What is the likelihood you would follow their prescribed treatment plan in the absence of a dialogue that acknowledges your beliefs and/or perception of the problem?

3.4 Health Literacy

Being mindful of a patient's health literacy is also paramount to the success of the clinical relationship and treatment outcomes.[4] Limited heath literacy impacts the ability to understand health information and to follow medical instructions, and ultimately determines health outcomes.[5] Since it varies so greatly among patients, it is beneficial to inquire how much they actually know about the diagnosis, surgery, procedure, or treatment plan they may be facing. This information will allow the caregiver to communicate in the most effective way and will promote shared treatment decision-making.

A patient's ability to comprehend presented information directly impacts the recall and follow-through of instructions.[6] Thus, certain techniques that encourage understanding through patient engagement have been found to enhance recall. These include open questioning, agenda setting, summarizing, and confirmation strategies such as the "teach-back" method wherein the patient demonstrates the skill that was taught (▶ Table 3.1).

Additionally, make a point to use a variety of media, including print materials that are at a suitable readability level and devoid of medical jargon. Materials not exceeding a fifth-grade reading level are suggested.[7] Encourage note taking on patient materials. Speak slowly, use plain language, and limit the amount of information provided during a single visit (▶ Fig. 3.1). Audiologist Cindy Pichler also suggests understanding the patient's learning style in order to enhance/maximize their comprehension of

---

Table 3.1 Techniques to enhance patient recall of information. Described in this table are patient-centered communication strategies to boost patient memory and subsequently improve treatment outcomes

Open questioning	Asking questions in a way that allows patients to share their concerns, such as "How?" and "Why?" "Tell me more…"
Agenda setting	Determining issues that are most important to the patient and creating a plan for what will be addressed during the visit
Confirming strategies	Requesting the patient repeat stated information in their own words, that is, "teach back"
Summarizing	Reviewing clinical data and instructions provided during the visit

---

Using plain language to promote understanding

- Discuss most important details first
- Break information into understandable chunks
- Use common vocabulary and define technical terms
- Speak in simple sentences, using the active voice

Data from Quick Guide to Health Literacy.
https://health.gov/communication/literacy/quickguide/factsbasic.htm (n.d.)

Fig. 3.1 Using plain language to promote understanding. Listed are communication guidelines for health care professionals that support patients' health literacy and encourage adherence of treatment plans.

information being presented. She recommends asking the patient the following questions to ascertain their preferred learning style:[8]

- Would you like to take notes or just listen?
- Do you want to see pictures of what is going on?
- Do you want to take these handouts and graphs that will explain what we will talk about?

When it comes to communicating with patients who have communication disorders, consider employing the following adaptations:[9]

- Identify the patient's preferred mode of communication.
- Include pauses to allow for more time to respond.
- Pose questions is a variety of ways.
- Use a white board/paper to communicate through words or illustrations.

3.5 Eliciting the Patient's Perspective

Perspective-taking includes inferring what may be going on in another's mind. Psychologist Nicholas Epley warns, however, that considering another's perspective is not a guarantee that you will be able to do it accurately.[10] This is particularly true in the absence of personal experience with the patient's situation. At best, trying to adopt another's perspective becomes an educated guess. Instead, Epley recommends asking questions and listening to help understand the other person's viewpoint, in other words, getting the other's perspective rather than taking it. Ultimately, it is through this kind of dialogue that we are able to discover the pathway to common ground.

Studies have shown that patients desire communication, partnership, and health promotion above any other "biomedical" aspect of the consultation.[11] Obtaining the patient's perspective is key to providing this kind of patient-centered care. It allows the caregiver to incorporate the patient's feelings and needs and to include them in the clinical decision-making process.[1] Taking this step will help garner trust because it demonstrates care and concern about their beliefs, wants, and fears.

Understanding and incorporating the patient's feelings and priorities into a therapy/treatment plan is paramount to achieving positive health outcomes.

Imagine you are going to buy a car and there are particular features that are extremely important to you (i.e., visibility, gas mileage, pairing smartphone, rear center seat lap/shoulder belt). How would you feel if you were never asked or given the opportunity to express the personal significance/necessity of those features with the salesperson? Is it likely you would buy a car from this person?

In the quest to gain the patient's perspective, discussion of the psychosocial issues surrounding the illness must be encouraged. Some fundamental areas to investigate include probable causes, hopes, fears, treatment expectations, acceptable risk levels, tolerable side effects, and therapeutic goals. To facilitate sharing and turn taking, caregivers can elicit information by asking open-ended questions such as the following:

- What are your concerns?
- What would you like to know?
- What do you think is causing your problem?
- How did it start?
- How is this affecting you?
- What do you feel could help you?

3.6 Power and Perspective-Taking

In his book, *To Sell is Human*, author Daniel H. Pink explains the importance of perspective-taking when attempting to move others. He specifically highlights its significance in health care, an arena where individuals are trying to influence, persuade, or modify the behaviors of others.[12] To that end, he reasons that the most accurate way to see another's point of view is by assuming that person is the one with the power. Research, in fact, supports that there is an inverse relationship between perspective-taking and social power.[13] In other words, by adopting the intention of "I am here to serve you" in lieu of "I am in charge here," the caregiver will become much more adept at seeing things from the patient's point of view.

Oftentimes, individuals who work on the front lines in service industries are unjustly perceived by others as having lower social power.

During the course of your day, boost your perspective-taking skills (and possibly your likeability) by assuming that you are not in a position of power as you interact with individuals who are providing services to you. As an example, observe an employee's tasks and work setting. Take note of the work volume, the necessity to multitask, or the speed and effort the job requires, and then make a comment to the individual demonstrating empathic acknowledgment of their employment situation.

3.7 Judgment Occludes Perspective

When we pass judgment, every piece of information that we process is interpreted through a tainted lens, and the ensuing emotions cloud our ability to make decisions based on facts. Accusatory thoughts of a patient's reckless, slothful, or self-inflicted behaviors make it difficult to isolate the behaviors from the person who displays them.

The Oath of Maimonides soundly instructs to "...never see in the patient anything but a fellow creature in pain."[14] Research on empathy has demonstrated that enhancing perspective taking coupled with a heightened value on the welfare of those unfamiliar to us can supersede any bias we may have.[15] Caregivers must therefore aspire to what humanistic psychologist Dr. Carl Rogers calls "unconditional positive regard." In carrying through this sympathetic act, we place personal opinions and judgments aside as to the worthiness of the patient and focus solely on healing the suffering.

3.8 Attunement and Perspective-Taking

Gaining another's perspective requires attunement or achieving harmony through awareness or responsivity.[16] More often than not, it is a wordless endeavor. Take for example the work of horse whisperers. They attune to their horses by using movement, body postures, and gestures that mimic the way horses communicate with one another. By communicating in the horses' "language," it calms them and promotes cooperation and bonding (i.e., harmony) between the equines and humans.

In a similar fashion, attunement in the medical setting requires reciprocal attention and gestures that demonstrate a degree of understanding between the caregiver and the patient. One way this can be achieved is via strategic mimicry—powerful, rapport-building nonverbal gestures that are intentionally used to match the patient's body language and vocal tone. For example, when meeting with a patient, you can mirror the position in which they are seated; use a similar size and type of gesturing, as well as adjust your energy level to that of the patient and their situation.

In the health care setting, strategic mimicry leads the patient to become more comfortable around the caregiver because they begin to feel they are like them. Through this exchange, mutual understanding unfolds, and a sense of connection arises.

> **Imagine This #4**   **i**
>
> Imagine you are in a hospital room, sitting by the bedside of a loved one who is getting ready to undergo a procedure. The room is quiet, and you are holding the loved one's hand when a staff member enters into the room. What type of vocal tone and intensity (loudness), mannerisms, and energy level would you hope that caregiver would exhibit to make your loved one feel the most understood and respected?

3.9 Empathy and Perspective-Taking

We can gain another's perspective by trying to understand and share feelings. Empathy, however, comes with two prerequisites. First, you have to care and, second, you must be able and willing to respond to the person's feelings.

3.9.1 Eye Contact and Empathy

Eye contact is a critical gateway to empathy, as feelings of compassion can be induced by simply witnessing a patient's emotional reaction. Neuroscience has revealed that when you make eye contact with another human being, it sends a signal to the brain that initiates both empathy and rapport.[17] In as few as 33 milliseconds of witnessing an emotion, the amygdala can read and identify it, allowing you to place yourself in the other person's "mental shoes" and begin to sense that same feeling within yourself.[18] Highly empathic individuals, because of their personal characteristics, have been shown to be particularly sensitive and responsive to the dynamic facial emotional expressions of others.[19]

3.9.2 Empathy and Facial Mimicry

Empathy can also be attained, in part, through mimicry. There is significant evidence that when individuals successfully mirror the physical behaviors that are tied to certain emotions, they are able to feel those same emotions themselves.[20] Psychologists James Laird and Katherine Lacasse, for example, report that, "In literally hundreds of experiments, when facial expressions, expressive behaviors, or visceral responses are induced, the corresponding feelings occur."[21] For instance, a caregiver may find themselves subconsciously mirroring the facial movements of the emotion displayed on the patient's face. If they are mimicking the outward display of sadness, they will start to adopt that same sorrowful state. Given the facial feedback theory, the movements will then trigger changes in their physiology, both in the body and the brain, which will in turn lead them to empathize with the emotion the patient is experiencing.[22]

Summary

Gaining the patient's perspective, including their knowledge, beliefs, and attitudes surrounding their illness, is essential to fully and respectfully addressing their needs. To be able to see the patient's situation through their eyes, however, calls upon the use of verbal and nonverbal communication that is open-minded and attuned to the patient. In doing so, the caregiver can demonstrate understanding and acceptance that will ultimately build their coveted trust in them.

References

[1] Stewart M. Towards a global definition of patient centred care. BMJ. 2001; 322(7284):444–445

[2] Kohli N, Dalal AK. Culture as a factor in causal understanding of illness: a study of cancer patients. Psychol Dev Soc J. 1998; 10(2):115–129

[3] Gerteis M, Edgman-Levitan S, Daley J, Delbanco T, eds. Through the patients' eyes: understanding and promoting patient-centered care. San Francisco, CA: Jossey-Bass; 1993

[4] Wynia MK, Osborn CY. Health literacy and communication quality in health care organizations. J Health Commun. 2010; 15 Suppl 2:102–115

[5] Kountz DS. Strategies for improving low health literacy. Postgrad Med. 2009; 121(5):171–177

[6] Laws MB, Lee Y, Taubin T, Rogers WH, Wilson IB. Factors associated with patient recall of key information in ambulatory specialty care visits: Results of an innovative methodology. https://www.ncbi.nlm.nih.gov/pubmed/29389994. Published 2018. Accessed November 8, 2018

[7] Villaire M, Mayer G. Low health literacy: the impact on chronic illness management. Prof Case Manag. 2007; 12(4):213–216, quiz 217–218

[8] Pichler CB. Effective patient communication. ASHA Lead. 2010; 15(4):5

[9] Blackstone SW, Beukelman DR, Yorkston KM. Patient-provider communication roles for speech-language pathologists and other health care professionals. San Diego, CA: Plural Publishing; 2015

[10] Epley N. Mindwise: how we understand what others think, believe, feel and want. London: Penguin Books; 2015

[11] Little P, Everitt H, Williamson I, et al. Preferences of patients for patient centred approach to consultation in primary care: observational study. BMJ. 2001; 322(7284):468–472

[12] Pink DH. To sell is human: the surprising truth about persuading, convincing, and influencing others. New York, NY: Penguin Group; 2012

[13] Markman A. Power, status, and perspective-taking. https://www.psychologytoday.com/us/blog/ulterior-motives/201606/power-status-and-perspective-taking. Published 2016. Accessed September 3, 2018

[14] Wikipedia. Oath of maimonides. https://en.m.wikipedia.org/wiki/Oath_of_Maimonides. Published 2017. Accessed April 20, 2017

[15] Riess H. The science of empathy. J Patient Exp. 2017; 4(2):74–77

[16] Merriam-Webster. Attune. https://www.merriam-webster.com/dictionary/attune. Accessed August 12, 2017

[17] Achor S. The happiness advantage: the seven principles that fuel success and performance at work. New York, NY: Crown Publishing Group; 2010

[18] Goleman D. Social intelligence. New York, NY: Bantam; 2006

[19] Rymarczyk K, Żurawski Ł, Jankowiak-Siuda K, Szatkowska I. Emotional empathy and facial mimicry for static and dynamic facial expressions of fear and disgust. Front Psychol. 2016; 7:1853

[20] Söderkvist S, Ohlén K, Dimberg U. How the experience of emotion is modulated by facial feedback. J Nonverbal Behav. 2018; 42(1):129–151

[21] Laird JD, Lacasse K. Bodily influences on emotional feelings: accumulating evidence and extensions of William James's theory of emotion. Emot Rev. 2013; 6(1):27–34

[22] Ekman P. Emotions revealed: recognizing faces and feelings to improve communication and emotional life. New York, NY: St. Martin's Griffin; 2007

Chapter 4

Addressing the Patient with the Intention to Bond

4 Addressing the Patient with the Intention to Bond

Abstract
This chapter offers the reader many fundamental skills to help patients feel at ease and connected to the caregiver within a short period of time. It begins by examining the pivotal role of intention in promoting therapeutic communication with patients. Next, it describes the social nuances of a caregiver–patient interaction. This includes the way the staff member introduces themself, addresses the patient, interacts with family, displays cultural sensitivity and "reads" the room. Specifically, this chapter delves into the importance of key aspects of that first meeting, including a pleasant facial expression, appropriate eye contact, and the just-right handshake. Making a good first impression is a critical step in bonding with patients. Moreover, the quality of the first encounter lays the groundwork for positive future interactions by establishing a foundation of mutual trust, care, and respect.

Keywords: positive first impression, therapeutic communication, caregiver–patient interaction, cultural sensitivity, communication strategies, connecting with patients

Attitude is a choice. Happiness is a choice. Optimism is a choice. Kindness is a choice. Giving is a choice. Respect is a choice. Whatever choice you make makes you. Choose wisely.
Roy T. Bennett

4.1 Eunice's Story

"Eunice!" That's what she called out to get my attention. I started shuffling my magazine, trying to close it as quick as I could, so I could join the young lady who I presume was a nursing assistant. She told me her name, but I can't remember it. I was trying to get past the fact that she called me by my first name.

The lady said, "Come this way," and just started marching ahead without as much as a look back at me. It was a long walk to our room—a left turn, then a right turn—and with each step all I could think of was how this was all going to turn out for me. When we finally got to the room, the nursing assistant told me to head over to the scale. Well I started moving in that direction, but when I saw her take a seat at a computer with her back facing me, I stopped dead in my tracks. I'm thinking, "She wants me to stand on the scale while she asks me questions?" So I just stood next to the examining table instead. At first, I was feeling awkward, but then I felt really put off by how I was being treated.

When the questions were done, we trudged over to that dreaded scale. I knew for sure I had put on a few pounds since my last visit. I could feel my heart thumping in my chest, and I decided to just avoid looking at the scale as I got on.

Then, the nursing assistant brought out the blood pressure cuff. Now why in the world would someone take your blood pressure right after you have just been on a scale? I mean, I was at my tipping point—and right on cue, she had the nerve to ask me, "Is your blood pressure always this high?"

4.2 About First Impressions

Making a good first impression is a critical step in bonding with clients and patients, and the quality of that initial encounter will lay the groundwork for positive future interactions. Oftentimes, there is only a brief window of opportunity to make the individual feel comfortable and cared for. In fact, most people in a worried state, like patients, will judge whether you are a caring person within 30 seconds of meeting you.[1] Moreover, once a person has reached a verdict, it is extremely difficult to change their mind.[2]

Imagine This #1	i
Imagine someone you have met in the past that you seemed to instantly like or dislike. What were the verbal or nonverbal behaviors of the individual that made you form the opinion so quickly?	

Accordingly, every social nuance of a clinical interaction requires careful examination. The way the caregiver introduces themself, addresses the patient, and uses nonverbal cues are among the communicative behaviors to consider when attempting to make a positive first impression. Outlined below are some of the foundational skills to help those we care for feel comfortable and connected within a short amount of time.

4.3 Creating a Positive First Impression

4.3.1 Clarify Your Intention toward Your Patients

When it comes to promoting therapeutic communication with clients and patients, intention is at the very root. This leaning of the heart is reflected in the manner in which the caregiver approaches the patient and dictates the level of communication at which they function (▶ Fig. 4.1).

Without conscious awareness, a caregiver's predisposition toward their job and patients are expressed in their nonverbal communication. For this reason, it is critical to ponder the following questions related to intention:

- Do I want to serve?
- Do I respect and care about my patients?
- Do I want my clients to like and trust me?
- Do I want to provide a notably good experience?

If the answers to these questions are "yes," then your intentions will be reflected in a compassionate vocal tone, facial expression, and body language and will promote communication that is therapeutic. In contrast, if the responses to these questions are "no" or ambivalent, the verbal and nonverbal behaviors that spring forth may become an obstacle to the patient's healing.[3]

Good Intentions, but Bad Life Circumstances

Clearly, even when we have good intentions and desire to be an agent of healing, our personal life circumstances can at times be emotionally burdensome. The resultant feelings can color our vocal tone and manifest in our body language—each negatively impacting our ability to connect with patients. In such cases, a conscious choice must

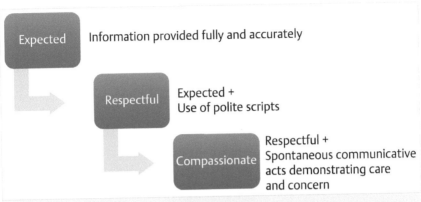

Fig. 4.1 Levels of communication in health care. This figure illustrates the progression of patient-centered communication from informational to respectful to the ultimate goal of communicating with kindness.

be made to put the patient first and attempt to present as kind, compassionate, and empathetic in spite of how we may be feeling on the inside. It is a noble act, and one that many health care heroes make every day.

Imagine This #2

Imagine a grumpy Snow White at Disney World. She would not stay employed for long. Part of this character actor's job, regardless of how she may be feeling inwardly, is to smile broadly and embrace the young children, as well as happily pose for pictures with them. For hours, she must walk around delighting her young audience. The present adults are aware that she is not superhumanly animated and carefree. On the contrary, she must consciously choose to appear that way in order to contribute to the children's joyous experience at the park (and to keep her employment).

When have you been personally challenged to present with a pleasant demeanor in spite of how you were truly feeling? If you had not chosen to be agreeable, how would it have affected the situation and the people around you?

4.4 Be Aware of Cultural Differences

Culture shapes how patients act and their expectations of how health care professionals should engage with them. Some cultural norms define gender, social, and family roles, as well as attitudes toward authority, displays of emotion, and personal space.[4] Other norms may apply to taboos about nudity and sexuality, in addition to hygienic and dietary practices.[4]

It is essential to be able to respond appropriately to individuals of varied cultures and diversities in order to promote mutual respect and trust. To this end, ask the patient directly if there are any cultural considerations for addressing and treating them.[5] Helpful resources can also be found on the internet that include information on patient care, meals, hospital attire, communication, rituals, and end-of-life care pertaining to a wide variety of cultures.

4.5 Learn to Read the Room

In the medical setting, caregivers face complex social interactions with individuals they may be encountering for the first time. Entering through the door, one does not know what the atmosphere in the room will be like. There may be crying, arguing, laughing, complaining, accusatory speech, calmness, hysterics, etc. To connect and respond appropriately to the patient's needs requires not only attending to his state, but also adapting one's social behaviors based on the circumstances and people surrounding them.

As you attempt to "read" the room, you are discerning the patient's situation at that moment in time. By using your senses, you can gather information like, "How does this person before me seem to be feeling? What kind of day is he having? Is this person feeling supported? What is the overall vibe in the room?"

Once you piece together the social information, you can modify your behavior accordingly. If the mood is somber, hopeful, or jubilant, you can adjust to an appropriate energy level and demeanor that reflects proper regard and understanding.

Imagine This #3 i

Imagine a health care professional who you, or someone you love, fully trust. What communication behaviors do they use to signal honesty, transparency, and directness?

4.6 Have a Pleasant Facial Expression

Dale Carnegie, author of *How to Win Friends and Influence People*, once said that the expression one wears on one's face is far more important than the clothes one wears on one's back.[6] This is particularly true in the health care setting as patients routinely form quick opinions about their caregivers based on facial expression. In fact, research reveals it takes only one-tenth of a second to form an impression of a stranger from their face.[7] The bottom line: make sure the first facial expression your patient witnesses is a pleasant one because it plays a significant role in how they perceive you and, ultimately, their willingness to trust and be open with you.

Take Action #1

From time to time, an individual will say, "People tell me I look mad even when I'm not." Are you aware of the way you look when your face is completely at rest? To find out, completely relax all of the muscles in your face and take a selfie. Next, continue to keep your facial muscles relaxed, but this time open up your eye area by raising your eyebrows slightly and then take another selfie. Compare the two pictures and note how just a small modification to your facial expression can make a vast difference in how you present to others.

The act of smiling, in particular, has been shown to promote cooperation in situations requiring mutual trust.[8] Even when we do not feel like it, smiling is a gift we can choose to give our clients and patients. When the intention behind the smile is to be kind and welcoming, it is perceived by the viewer as authentic. The more genuine the smile, the more strongly it predicts judgments about the trustworthiness of the person who is smiling.[8]

4.7 Make and Maintain Appropriate Eye Contact

Eye contact with your patient is a critical means of building connection. In most cultures (be aware of differences), it communicates respect by signifying that they have your full attention.

Additionally, by maintaining eye contact with the patient, you are showing that you are confident, trustworthy, and competent. Not enough eye contact, on the other hand, may signal to the patient the exact opposite, or that information is being withheld. As a result, their faith in you diminishes.

Imagine This #4

Imagine a time when you have shaken someone's hand and you had an immediate visceral response. Did the experience lead you to feel differently toward that person?

4.8 Shake Your Patient's Hand

When appropriate, upon greeting and parting, use the "just-right" handshake to signal interest, respect, and sincerity. To that end, avoid offering limp fingers, squeezing too hard, and using only the finger tips. Each will leave a poor impression that is literally and figuratively hard to shake. Instead, keep your palm vertical, meet the web (contour between the thumb and index finger) of your hand with the web of the other person's hand, and give the same pressure you are receiving.[9]

Make sure to establish eye contact as you shake hands. When performed together, they present an opportune moment to connect with the patient, as opposed to carrying out a simple formality (▶ Table 4.1).

Take Action #2

A proper handshake instills confidence and trustworthiness and creates rapport. Make sure yours is communicating the right message by soliciting the opinion of someone you hold in high regard.

Practice using the just-right handshake described earlier. Always remember to make eye contact while you are shaking hands.

Table 4.1 Character traits associated with handshake types. Emphasized are the negative impressions formed by improper handshakes

Type	Association
Too soft	Weakness
Too hard	Aggressiveness/dominance
Finger tips only	Insecurity
Just right	Competence/trustworthiness

4.9 Introduce Yourself

Patients come in contact with a variety of professionals across settings. Introducing yourself and describing in what way you will try to help is polite and goes a long way toward making the patient feel comfortable.

4.10 Ask Patients How They Would Like to Be Addressed

Addressing clients and patients the wrong way can lead to upset.[10] Many are not opposed to being called by their first name, but some find it disrespectful. The best practice is to ask them directly how they prefer to be addressed.[11]

Hearing one's name is particularly relevant for patients who may experience a deep sense of anonymity and loss of identity in the hospital setting. In other health care settings, it is equally significant because they may be internalizing strong feelings of vulnerability and powerlessness in the face of their illness or disability. The sound of their name can help restore a sense of self and assist them in feeling acknowledged and valued. For this reason, also make a point to use patients' names multiple times during an encounter, as it activates areas of the brain associated with the self, including self-judgment and evaluation of personal qualities.[12]

Take Action #3

Dale Carnegie once shared: "Remember that a person's name is to that person the sweetest and most important sound in any language."

Today, make a point to look at a service provider's (i.e., bank teller, cashier, librarian) name badge. Along with eye contact and a smile, use the individual's name upon greeting and parting. Continue to practice this courtesy until it becomes a habit that you enact with every person you encounter. Notice the positive reaction you get from others just from performing this simple act of acknowledgment.

4.11 Become Acquainted with the Patient's Story

Your intention toward the patient dictates the verbal choices you make during conversation and reflects whether or not you value them as an individual. One way to show the patient that you care for them as a human being is by getting acquainted with their personal story.

Soliciting the patient's story promotes empathy and human connection. While they share, demonstrate you are listening by using acknowledging behaviors, making comments and following up with questions. To strengthen your bond, try to identify and express areas you may have in common, such as place of birth, nationality, hobbies, favorite sport's teams, etc. In the hospital setting, be alert to patients' pictures, flowers, balloons, stuffed animals, etc. By commenting on these personal items, you will highlight the affection and support of loved ones as well as signal to the patient that you appreciate them as a person.

> ### Take Action #4 ✔
>
> John Dewy, famous American philosopher, believed that the most profound urge in human nature is the desire to be important. The fulfillment of this longing, however, can be difficult for clients and patients to achieve in the health care setting when focus is too narrowly placed on the patient's clinical status and not enough on the personhood.
>
> Consider freely giving the gift of honest appreciation to someone today. At work, comment on a colleague who is excelling or making a difference by their actions. At home, point out to a loved one something positive they did that was helpful or meaningful. If you are currently working in a health care setting, affirm the patient or client's self-worth by illuminating something about the individual that makes them unique and special.

Summary

The first few minutes of an initial encounter play a prophetic role in the relationship between the caregiver and the patient. When the caregiver approaches the patient with a desire to bond and employs the many communication strategies that leave a positive first impression, a solid foundation is laid for a partnership based on mutual care, trust, and respect.

References

[1] Greenberger LS. What to say when things get tough: business communication strategies for winning people over when they're angry, worried and suspicious of everything you say. New York, NY: McGraw-Hill Education; 2013

[2] Schafer J. Why our negative first impressions are so powerful. https://www.psychologytoday.com/us/blog/let-their-words-do-the-talking/201412/why-our-negative-first-impressions-are-so-powerful. Published 2014. Accessed December 12, 2017

[3] Ambady N, Koo J, Rosenthal R, Winograd CH. Physical therapists' nonverbal communication predicts geriatric patients' health outcomes. Psychol Aging. 2002; 17(3):443–452

[4] Gerteis M, Edgman-Levitan S, Daley J, Delbanco T, eds. Through the patients' eyes: understanding and promoting patient-centered care. San Francisco, CA: Jossey-Bass; 1993

[5] The Joint Commission. Advancing effective communication, cultural competence, and patient- and family-centered care: a roadmap for hospitals. Oakbrook Terrace, IL: The Joint Commission; 2010

[6] Carnegie D. How to win friends & influence people. New York, NY: Pocket Books; 2007

[7] Willis J, Todorov A. First impressions: making up your mind after a 100-ms exposure to a face. Psychol Sci. 2006; 17(7):592–598

[8] Centorrino S, Djemai E, Hopfensitz A, Milinski M, Seabright P. Honest signaling in trust interactions: smiles rated as genuine induce trust and signal higher earning opportunities. Evol Hum Behav. 2015; 36(1):8–16

[9] Pease A. Body language, the power is in the palm of your hands | Allan Pease | TEDxMacquarieUniversity. https://m.youtube.com/watch?v=ZZZ7k8cMA-4. Published November 17, 2013. Accessed December 9, 2018

[10] Merlino J. Service fanatics: how to build superior patient experience the Cleveland clinic way. New York, NY: McGraw-Hill Education; 2015

[11] Agency for Healthcare Research and Quality. Guide to patient and family engagement in hospital quality and safety. http://www.ahrq.gov/professionals/systems/hospital/engagingfamilies/index.html. Published 2013. Accessed January 4, 2018

[12] Carmody DP, Lewis M. Brain activation when hearing one's own and others' names. Brain Res. 2006; 1116 (1):153–158

Chapter 5

Employing Positive Body Language

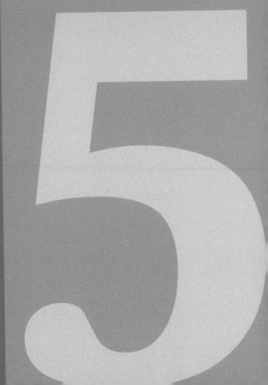

5 Employing Positive Body Language

Abstract

This chapter explores the role of nonverbal communication in promoting patient trust and respect while subsequently boosting patient satisfaction. Highlighted are positive body language cues (postures and gestures, eye contact, facial expression, proximity, and touch) that can be used during patient–provider interactions. Each demonstrates openness and compassion and ultimately facilitates connection. Furthermore, this chapter probes the vital role of intention, as well as emotion, in influencing our non-verbal behaviors. Caregivers who have positive attitudes and beliefs toward their patients and who can regulate their emotions will involuntarily exhibit nonverbal behaviors that demonstrate kindness and compassion. For this reason, it is necessary for health care providers to achieve a high level of self-awareness regarding this mind-body interplay and how it manifests in their body language. Additionally, this chapter investigates the wordless messages the patient may be sending. By learning to read these signals, perceptive caregivers can better understand and serve the patient's physical and emotional needs.

Keywords: nonverbal communication, nonverbal behaviors, patient satisfaction, body language, compassion, patient–provider interaction, proximity, touch, mind–body

Too often we underestimate the power of a touch, a smile, a kind word, a listening ear, an honest compliment, or the smallest act of caring, all of which have the potential to turn a life around.

Leo Buscaglia

5.1 Jerry's Story

My father needed a new urologist, so I did some research and found one that had really good reviews. When I took dad to the first visit, he was afraid. He was physically weak and feeling very anxious. It didn't help that the office was in this imposing building. When we got up to the doctor's floor, a nurse greeted us and led us to the back. Now she was amazing—she made eye contact, smiled, and chitchatted with my father as we walked. I could see my dad engaging with her, even smiling. Some of his anxiety was melting away right before my eyes and his mood certainly perked up.

Oftentimes when I take my dad to see different specialists, I will act as his caretaker and provide them with his history. In the end, they always seem to focus on me more than my dad, even though he is cognitively just fine. This new urologist Dr. U, however, was different. He made sure to give dad plenty of attention. On his rolling stool, he would pivot back and forth between my dad and his computer, always turning right back to talk to him and look at him eye to eye. Sure, he would glance my way and engage with me too, but through his body language he made it clear that my father was his focus of attention and the one making the choices.

Being older, dad had speech that was just naturally slower. Dr. U always gave him the space he needed to express himself. He also took the time to verbally acknowledge and affirm that my dad's situation was not easy. That meant a lot to both of us.

What I most remember about Dr. U was his great eye contact and the way he smiled at dad. His whole manner was calming, including his tone of voice. Even when he spoke, it was at just the right speed. He never seemed rushed. He would always wind up saying things two and three times over to make sure dad understood. My father never felt like he was being bullied to do anything. He always made dad feel like he had a say in the treatment.

Basically, everything Dr. U did showed that he cared. He saw dad as a whole person, and not just this urinary tract system that needed to be treated. We saw Dr. U a few times over a 6-month period, and he was consistently the same: caring and respectful.

5.2 About Nonverbal Communication

Across all fields of employment, what matters most to employees and the people they serve is to feel at ease, acknowledged, and affirmed in their relationships.[1] While dialogue plays an important part in forging this interconnection, the nonverbal realm of communication is where most of these goals are achieved.

Nonverbal communication is comprised of both body language and vocal tone. Body language encompasses our body postures, gestures, proximity (nearness in space), and facial expressions, whereas vocal tone refers to the pitch and inflection we use during speech, along with our vocal loudness, pacing, and pausing (▶ Fig. 5.1).

Research has confirmed that nonverbal signals carry a significantly greater impact than the words expressed during conversation.[2] How does this impact the caregiver's delivery of effective, compassionate communication? It demands placing a premium on nonverbal behaviors that engender trust and respect, and in turn, lead to connection. At the same time, it requires picking up on the wordless messages the patient is sending to better understand and serve their needs.

Imagine This #1	i

The nonverbal realm of communication is where we draw most of our information when we communicate.

For instance, imagine you have just purchased a new article of clothing, and you would like to know what a loved one thinks of it. Would you rely more on the individual's verbal comments or on the way they look and sound when providing the feedback?

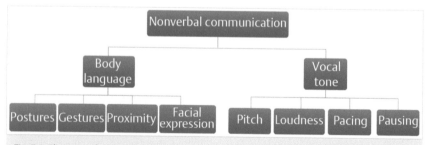

Fig. 5.1 Elements of nonverbal communication. Listed are the subcomponents of body language and vocal tone.

5.3 Our Nonverbal Language

When it comes to interpersonal communication, it is important to recognize that there are actually two conversations that are taking place. The first is the one we are cognizant of, which is the words we are saying. The second is the one that often happens without our conscious awareness, the nonverbal communication.

> **Take Action #1**
>
> We are communicating at all times. Even in complete silence our bodies are continuously sending messages out to others.
>   Choose a moment today and create a mental inventory of what your body looks like in that instant. Reflect on what your body language may be "saying" to others. Use information regarding body language signals from this chapter, as well as from Chapter 2.

- How are you holding your head? Is your chin level or tucked into your neck?
- Is there muscle tension in your face that may be reflected in your jaw, lips, and eyebrows?
- Is your breathing deep or shallow?
- If you are speaking with someone, where is your torso angled?
- Are your shoulders pulled back or slumping forward?
- How are you holding your hands? Are they clasped, clenched, fidgeting, or simply lying flat and side by side?
- Are your arms by your side or crossed in front of your body?
- How are your legs resting—side by side, crossed over, or locked at the ankles? Are your feet still or jiggling?

As with other aspects of communication, it is our intention that informs our nonverbal communication.[3] Caregivers who have positive attitudes and beliefs toward their patients will involuntarily exhibit nonverbal behaviors that demonstrate kindness and compassion. In fact, merely the desire to relieve a patient's suffering will be reflected in much of our body language.

> **Imagine This #2**
>
> Imagine a caregiver who you perceive to be kind and caring. How does the individual communicate warmth via body language signals? What is the individual's typical facial expression like?

5.3.1 The Mind–Body Connection

Just as intention is reflected in nonverbal communication, so too is emotion. Essentially, we experience an emotion, and without our conscious awareness it is displayed via our body language and vocal tone. Facial expressions, hand gestures, postures, and vocal elements, therefore, communicate to your patients a tremendous amount about how you are feeling and about your state of mind. See ▶ Video 1.1. For this reason, caregivers must be alert to whether this mind–body interplay is having a positive or negative affect on their patient interactions (▶ Fig. 5.2).

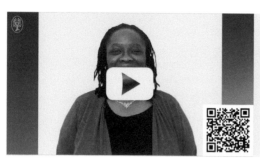

Video 1.1 Using Positive Body Language During Patient-Provider Communication and video URL: https://www.thieme.de/de/q.htm?p=opn/cs/19/11/10686240-a2227929

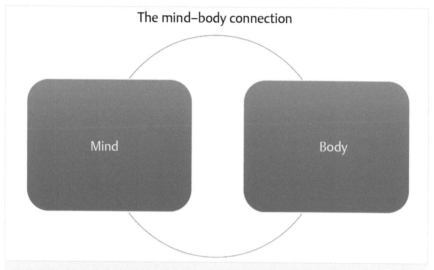

Fig. 5.2 The mind–body connection. This figure depicts the communication feedback loop that exists between the mind and the body.

5.3.2 Postures and Gestures

Given the mind–body connection, assuming certain body postures influences how we think and feel, and in turn affects how the people around us think and feel. Take, for example, the caregiver who exudes confidence by standing tall, with shoulders back, stomach in, and head up. They not only feel self-assured but are perceived by their patients as competent and trustworthy (▶ Fig. 5.3).[4]

In addition to feelings of self-assurance, enacting certain postures and gestures can promote connection with patients by communicating openness and authenticity. Postures may include any of the following: a torso turned toward the patient and leaning forward, arms and legs uncrossed,[5] a hand held over the heart, head tilting, and head nods. Additionally, leaning the torso forward signals engagement and interest (▶ Fig. 5.4 and ▶ Fig. 5.5).[4]

The open palm is a particularly strong signal of openness, indicating "I have nothing to hide" or "You can trust me." Interestingly, simply displaying an open palm can encourage the patient you are speaking with to be more open with you as well (▶ Fig. 5.6).[6]

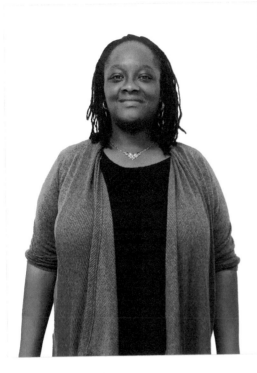

Fig. 5.3 Confident body postures communicate competence and trustworthiness.

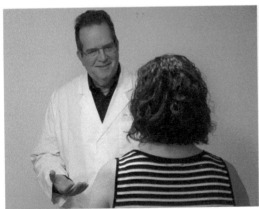

Fig. 5.4 An example of open-body posture.

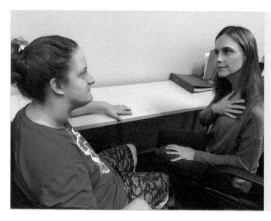

Fig. 5.5 Body language that promotes connection.

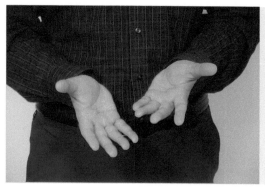

Fig. 5.6 The open palm gesture signals sincerity.

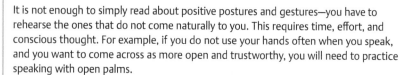

Take Action #2

It is not enough to simply read about positive postures and gestures—you have to rehearse the ones that do not come naturally to you. This requires time, effort, and conscious thought. For example, if you do not use your hands often when you speak, and you want to come across as more open and trustworthy, you will need to practice speaking with open palms.

At some point today, commit to speaking part of the time with open palms as you converse with another person. Continue to practice the gesture during other conversations until it becomes second nature to you.

However, at times, we may desire to appear as open and compassionate, but our body language does not align with that intention due to habitual postures. For example, some of us cover our mouth when we speak, cross our arms when we are standing, stare at the floor, lock our ankles, fiddle with our cuticles—all out of habit. In these cases, it is necessary to extinguish those habits by purposefully practicing positive, open body postures and making them an established way of how we present to our patients.

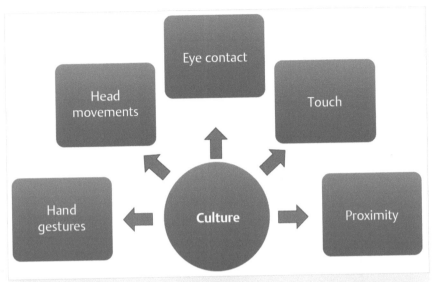

Fig. 5.7 Influence of culture on body language. Depicted are the nonverbal signals that require cultural sensitivity.

Hand Signals

While people around the world share most of the basic communication signals, it is crucial to be attentive to the various cultural nuances of gestures, eye contact, facial expressions, proximity, and touch.

For example, in the case of hand signals, the "OK" sign and the "thumbs up" sign (which are often used in the health care setting) carry diverse meanings across nationalities. It is wise to keep in mind with whom you are communicating as using those gestures can be insulting to some cultures (▶ Fig. 5.7).[6]

5.3.3 Facial Expression

Your countenance directly influences the patient's attitude toward you and how they respond to you. A positive facial expression helps patients feel comfortable in your presence and promotes a willingness to trust and to be open with you. As a rule, opened eyes, raised eyebrows, and smiling all reflect receptivity and communicate warmth (▶ Fig. 5.8).

It has been shown that facial cues reflecting care, concern, and empathy improve physical and cognitive health in some patients.[7] When it comes to flashing a smile, for example, the patient is likely to smile at you too, because humans unconsciously mimic the actions and facial expressions of others.[8] As the patient turns up the corners of their mouth, positive feelings are induced. In contrast, when the provider does not smile, or looks away, decreases in functioning have been found to occur (▶ Fig. 5.9).[7]

Also noteworthy is how patients are astute observers due to their heightened state. They are always analyzing facial expressions to gather information, attempting to discern either hope or concern from the caregiver's expression.[9]

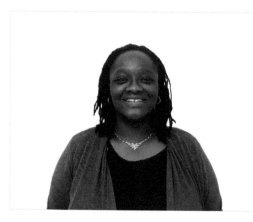

Fig. 5.8 A pleasant facial expression communicates friendliness.

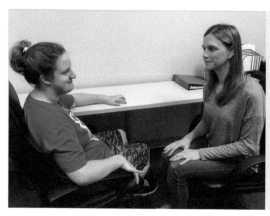

Fig. 5.9 Smiling, a powerful facial cue that invokes feelings of trust.

Dr. Edward E. Rosenbaum, author of *A Taste of My Own Medicine*, describes a personal encounter with one of his doctors: "But then he did something that comforted me. He smiled. He was the first doctor who had done that. I knew that he was only being pleasant, but it gave me some hope. I realized that I was looking for any sign that everything was all right."

5.3.4 Eye Contact

When possible, ensure your gaze occurs at the patients' eye level (▶ Fig. 5.10). Caregivers who speak with their patients face to face are perceived to be more compassionate and professional, as well as to have better communication skills.[10] Accordingly, choosing to sit down is a physical motion that conveys a great deal of information to patients. It is a silent cue communicating equality and acceptance, and signals that you have time for them.[11] Conversely, remaining standing for the entire visit while the patient is sitting, or reclined, may be subliminally interpreted as, "I am above you." He may begin to feel intimidated, particularly if you are already perceived as an authority figure.

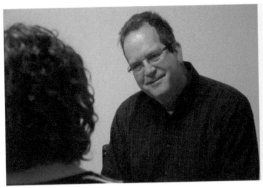

Fig. 5.10 Eye contact at the patient's visual level demonstrates respect.

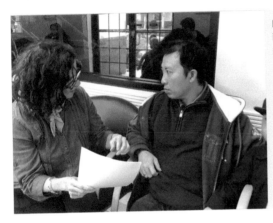

Fig. 5.11 Establishing close interpersonal space can be perceived as supportive.

5.3.5 Proximity

Proxemics is the study of space as it relates to communication between people. The amount of space necessary to feel comfortable during an interaction varies between cultures and from individual to individual; and personal preference is made clear through body language cues (▶ Fig. 5.11).

In the medical setting, proximity is particularly relevant when you are discussing sensitive issues that affect patients. Establishing close interpersonal space, for instance, lends intimacy to the encounter. Also, the primitive emotional regions of our brains become activated, which may assist in better understanding what the patient is feeling.[12] Additionally, remaining close signals to the patient that there is someone else on his side to support him. Distance, on the other hand, may lead to disconnection, leaving the patient to feel like he is on his own to confront whatever lies ahead.

5.3.6 Touch

Touch is a powerful nonverbal gesture used to connect with others, and its influence can be seen across a variety of work settings. Savvy restaurant servers, for example, employ it to their advantage, earning higher tips if they pat their customers when handing them the bill.[4] Successful salespeople also capitalize on touch, using a light, 3-second elbow touch to quickly bond with their clients.[6]

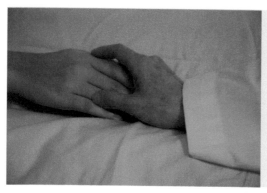

Fig. 5.12 Touch can be healing to the patient.

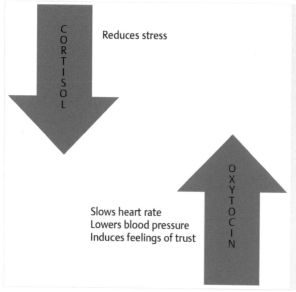

Fig. 5.13 The benefits of touch. This figure demonstrates the impact of touch on hormones that positively influence well-being.

C
O
R
T
I
S
O
L

Reduces stress

O
X
Y
T
O
C
I
N

Slows heart rate
Lowers blood pressure
Induces feelings of trust

In the medical arena, a kind touch can significantly contribute to a patient's healing process (▶ Fig. 5.12). It leads to the release of oxytocin, which in turn lowers blood pressure, decreases cortisol (the stress hormone), increases pain tolerance,[13] and induces feelings of trust. For this reason, touch is often used to calm emotions or to serve as a reminder for the patient to regain composure (▶ Fig. 5.13).

Rubbing and patting are two forms of touch employed to show sympathy or to communicate support.[14] Touch can also convey positive emotions like care and compassion and can be an empathetic response to something that is uncomfortable or perhaps difficult to relay with words. Just a brief tap to the hand or arm lets clients and patients feel acknowledged and that they are not alone.

5.3.7 When Body Language and Words Are Out of Sync

Patients discern the health care professional's attitudes and thoughts by synthesizing information that comes in through their senses. Subconsciously, they perceive and interpret nonverbal cues, like facial expression, eye contact, vocal pitch changes, proximity, postures, and gestures. When these nonverbal elements are congruent, or in agreement with what is being said, the same message is communicated simultaneously and the speaker comes across as authentic and trustworthy.

In some instances, however, a contradiction between the caregiver's words and body language occurs. Hence, the words do not mask the caregiver's real intention, and their body language exposes the truth. For example, if they say, "How are you feeling today?" and the patient does not see a matching expression of interest or concern on their face, then they have essentially revealed their actual sentiment—apathy. In time, this incongruence between body language and verbal expression can erode a patient's confidence and trust in the health care professional.

Imagine This #3 　　　　　　　　　　　　　　　　　　　　　　**i**

Imagine a time when someone said something to you and it was not corroborated in their body language. What were the signals that did not align with the words you heard? What feeling did you get?

5.4 Nonverbal Behaviors to Avoid

There are certain nonverbal behaviors that hinder communication with patients (▶ Fig. 5.14). Crossed arms, legs, and feet, as well as hands in the pockets can all be perceived as barriers during an interaction. Other behaviors that prevent connection include looking at a watch, drumming fingers, glancing at the door, or maintaining one hand on the doorknob or door frame. Each suggests the caregiver may be in a hurry and has little or no time for the patient.

Another obstacle to communication occurs when the caregiver engages with a computer or looks down to review records for an extended period of time. This act can lead the patient to feel uncomfortable, or even ignored. In this instance, the goal is to convey to the patient that your mutual interaction is more valuable than interfacing with a computer or managing paperwork. Consider employing some of these positive verbal and nonverbal strategies:

- Use small talk, coupled with affirming nonverbal behaviors to make the patient feel comfortable and cared for.
- If computer use is necessary, explain what it will be used for and for how long. When dialogue is required during computer use, momentarily stop typing to look at the patient while speaking.
- When engaging with a computer, ensure it is positioned in such a way as to involve the patient, and when appropriate, to allow the patient to look at the screen with you.

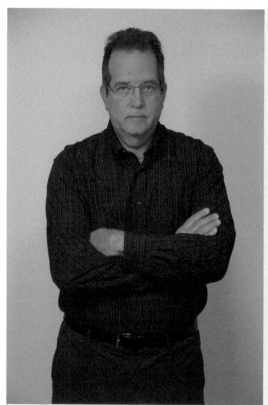

Fig. 5.14 Closed-body postures create a barrier to communication.

5.5 The Patients' Nonverbal Communication

Crossed arms, a head hanging low, monotone speech, and frequent pausing are just a few ways body language and vocal tone can speak louder than words about the patient's emotional condition (▶ Fig. 5.15). The caregiver's ability to pick up on a patient's nonverbal communication plays a significant role in the bonding process. If our desire is to treat "the whole patient" and to be conduits of healing, we must be aware of his nonverbal cues so we can attend to his emotional condition and not just his physical state. With that said, it calls upon an open heart for our senses to receive all the audible and inaudible messages directed our way.

In listening with our full body, we engage our unconscious and begin tuning into vital information we may have otherwise missed.[5] With mindful awareness, we can take notice of the patient's energy level, their use of eye contact, body language, facial expressions, vocal tone, etc., to ascertain the deeper meaning behind their nonverbal cues.

By deciphering patients' nonverbal cues, we can also begin to identify what they are truly thinking and feeling. We can glean important information like: Do they feel hopeful? Are they understanding me? Are they open to what I am saying? This nonverbal sensitivity directly influences the effectiveness of the caregiver's feedback and has been

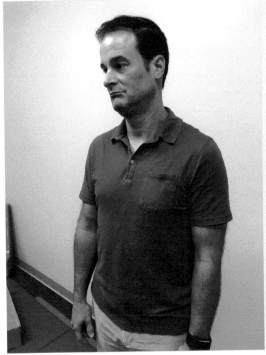

Fig. 5.15 A patient's nonverbal cues speak louder than words.

shown to significantly impact the interpersonal success between the health care provider and the patient in the clinical setting.[15]

Take Action #3

Reading patients'/clients' body language cues is critical as it improves our ability to be more sensitive to their feelings and emotions.

Practice increasing your body language acuity today. During each interaction with others, approach with the mindset that when you part you will be able to recall a nonverbal signal exhibited by your communication partner.

Summary

Patients form opinions about health care professionals based on how they feel during a mutual interaction, and that feeling is to a large extent linked to the staff member's nonverbal behaviors. Information pours in both consciously and subconsciously, leading to complex evaluations that are made very quickly as to what their caregiver thinks/feels about them. Thus, caregivers must achieve a high level of self-awareness in regard to their intention, body language, and vocal tone, ensuring they reflect authenticity, care, and trustworthiness.

At the same time, caregivers must also attend to their patients' nonverbal signals. By cuing into their silent messages, we can pick up on how the patients are feeling on the inside and use that information to effectively communicate to meet both their physical and emotional needs.

References

[1] Carnegie D. How to win friends & influence people. New York, NY: Pocket Books; 2007

[2] Reiman T. The power of body language: how to succeed in every business and social encounter. New York, NY: Pocket Books; 2009

[3] Meyers P, Nix S. As we speak: how to make your point and have it stick. New York, NY: Atria Paperback; 2012

[4] Goman CK. The nonverbal advantage: secrets and science of body language at work. San Francisco, CA: Berrett-Koehler Publishers, Inc.; 2008

[5] Morgan N. Trust me: four steps to authenticity and charisma. San Francisco, CA: Jossey-Bass; 2009

[6] Pease A, Pease B. The definitive book of body language. New York, NY: Bantam Books; 2006

[7] Ambady N, Koo J, Rosenthal R, Winograd CH. Physical therapists' nonverbal communication predicts geriatric patients' health outcomes. Psychol Aging. 2002; 17(3):443–452

[8] Riess H. The science of empathy. J Patient Exp. 2017; 4(2):74–77

[9] Rosenbaum EE. A taste of my own medicine: when the doctor is the patient. New York, NY: Random House; 1988

[10] Haider A, Tanco K, Epner M, et al. Physicians' compassion, communication skills, and professionalism with and without physicians' use of an examination room computer: a randomized clinical trial. JAMA Oncol. 2018; 4(6):879–881

[11] Deardorff J. Should doctors sit or stand. http://featuresblogs.chicagotribune.com/features_julieshealthclub/2010/04/should-doctors-sit-or-stand-.html Published 2010. Accessed June 11, 2015

[12] Beilock S. How the body knows its mind. London: Robinson; 2015

[13] Uvnas-Moberg K, Petersson M. Oxytocin, a mediator of anti-stress, well-being, social interaction, growth and healing. https://www.ncbi.nlm.nih.gov/pubmed/15834840. Published 2005. Accessed February 07, 2017

[14] Hertenstein MJ, Holmes R, McCullough M, Keltner D. The communication of emotion via touch. Emotion. 2009; 9(4):566–573

[15] Roter DL, Frankel RM, Hall JA, Sluyter D. The expression of emotion through nonverbal behavior in medical visits. Mechanisms and outcomes. J Gen Intern Med. 2006; 21 Suppl 1:S28–S34

Chapter 6

Listening with the Heart and the Mind

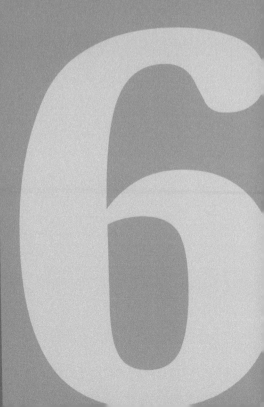

6 Listening with the Heart and the Mind

Abstract

This chapter details the essential verbal and nonverbal strategies used to signal to the patient that they are seen, heard, and valued. Some highlights include the use of open-bodied postures, acknowledging behaviors and statements, sharing the conversational floor, emotion labeling, and minimal encouragers. Additionally, this chapter describes methods to confirm the understanding of what the patient is communicating, including reflective listening and open-ended and clarifying questions. Engaging in active listening is a conscious, compassionate choice on the part of the caregiver and plays a pivotal role in the patient's healing process. The health care professional must have positive intentions toward the patient as well as a mindful state. This makes listening therapeutic. By attending verbally and nonverbally to patients, the caregiver is able to attune to their perspective by providing them the opportunity to share personal desires, beliefs, and fears. When patients are permitted to speak freely and feel understood, it is a gift that promotes connection and trust in the patient who requires healing of both the mind and the body.

Keywords: compassionate listening, active listening, healing process, verbal forms of active listening, nonverbal forms of active listening, patient's perspective, verbal strategies, nonverbal strategies, reflective listening, open-ended questions, clarifying questions

Listening is an attitude of the heart, a genuine desire to be with another which both attracts and heals.

J. Isham

6.1 Connie's Story

"Well you are obese, you need to lose 30 pounds." I kid you not; those were among the first words my new general practitioner doctor said to me. My extra weight was no news flash, but I certainly didn't need to be shamed like this by someone I had never met before. He then proceeded to lecture me on the necessity of working out and how "most middle-aged women don't know how to work out properly or have just decided they are too busy." I could feel my face burning red—but did he notice? Did he change his tone or tactics? Nope.

I began to try to explain how I worked out at least five times a week including running, yoga, step aerobics, body weight training, and exercise videos like Tracy Anderson, Nike, and others. I mentioned, however, that I have a history of back pain and had to quit running this past year. While I'm talking, he is nodding his head rapidly—basically telling me with his body to hurry up and finish what I was saying. He did not follow-up on the back issue, nor did he hear a word I had said, because he then repeats how I need to go to a gym and do weight training several times a week. Get this—he even offers me a coupon for a free trial to a gym!

So now I am beginning to think, not only does this doctor have problems hearing, but he has problems seeing too! Can he not see that my arms and legs are very toned, and that I'm only pudgy in the middle where I tend to keep weight? My heart is thumping wildly in my chest, and I decide to ask him if he knows what body weight training is.

Well, surprise, surprise—no response, just a mumbled brush off and a quick shift to how I may have sleep apnea—"a possible reason for your weight gain," he says. Not sure how he arrived at sleep apnea—nothing I had said to him gave any indication of a problem in that area.

6.2 About Compassionate Listening

Health conditions can be severe, chronic, painful, complex, and mysterious—invoking adverse emotions that can be as deleterious as the physical effects. Even mild ailments, like a lingering cold, may trigger feelings of sadness or hopelessness. A caregiver's compassionate listening, therefore, is a vital component to the patient's healing process. Allowing the patient to share about their condition and the emotions they are experiencing helps them to feel validated as a human being, and that they are not alone in their struggle. James R. Doty, neurosurgeon and founder of The Center for Compassion and Altruism Research and Education, explains his approach to patients who needed a listening ear: "I let each of them tell his or her story, and then I acknowledged my patients' struggles, their accomplishments, and their suffering. And in many cases, this relieved their pain more than any medication."[1]

Author Alene Nitzky, PhD, RN, describes listening as "what we do when we take the time to build a relationship with a patient."[2] It is a fundamental means of showing patients we care. True listening takes place when we put whatever we are thinking or doing on pause and focus solely on the individual in front of us. Nitzky asserts that health care providers who are fully engaged with their patients can pick up on important information beyond medical facts, like family members who are present, specific details about their lives, as well as goals for their health outcomes. By focusing on the individual, and not simply on their illness, the patient–provider relationship is strengthened.

Effective listening, however, is not an innate skill. It is a conscious, selfless choice that requires determination and practice. Below are key components of nonverbal and verbal active listening to begin exercising today.

6.3 Nonverbal Behaviors of Active Listening

6.3.1 Examine Your Intention

The first prerequisite of being a good listener is having a caring heart. The caregiver has to be able to see the patient as someone in need, and sincerely desire to ease his suffering. At the same time, it requires an awareness that listening style has the power to be either a conduit or an impediment to that person's healing.

6.3.2 Engage in Mindfulness

To feel validated, the patient must believe that they have your full attention when they are speaking to you. Therefore, an essential first step in active listening is establishing a mindful state. Buddhist monk Thich Nhat Hanh refers to it as "...letting go of judgment, returning to an awareness of the breath and the body, and bringing your full attention to what is around you."[3]

Being aware of what is going on within you is equally imperative. Simply ask yourself, "Am I in a state to take in information, or are my thoughts tangled up in other concerns?"

Imagine This #1

Have you ever been able to detect a time when someone has stopped listening to you, or the person's mind is on something else? What signals was the individual inadvertently sending. How did it make you feel?

Equally important is avoiding the temptation to formulate a response while listening to the patient. In his book, *The 7 Habits of Highly Effective People*,[4] Stephen Covey cautions: "Most people do not listen with the intent to understand; they listen with the intent to reply." Compassionate listening, by comparison, necessitates quieting the mind to fully take in the patient's perspective in lieu of focusing on a reply.

Imagine This #2

Imagine a time when you were having a conversation with someone, and while the individual was talking, you were trying to figure out what to say next. How was the quality of the conversation impacted since you had not given the person your full attention?

6.3.3 Use Appropriate Eye Contact

Using good eye contact not only demonstrates that you are paying attention but also places you in the best position for picking up on the client's nonverbal cues.

6.3.4 Adopt Open-Bodied Postures

Body postures and gestures signal to your patients whether you are listening and responsive to what they are saying.

Given the mind–body connection, an open body also reflects an open mind and vice versa. It not only facilitates perspective taking, but also research has demonstrated that we actually take in more information and retain it when we assume open body postures.[5]

6.3.5 Attend to the Patient's Body Language and Vocal Tone

See Chapter 5 under section: The Patients' Nonverbal Communication. The way patients use their bodies and voices signal how they are really feeling and will assist the caregiver in providing the most meaningful responses during conversation.

6.3.6 Employ Acknowledging Behaviors

In a world filled with indifference, any gesture, facial expression, or word that affirms another human being is a priceless gift. Such is the case with acknowledging behaviors. They communicate to the person with whom you are speaking that they are seen, heard, and valued. It may be a look of sadness precipitating something that was shared, a hand placed over the heart, or, most commonly, a head nod.

Nodding your head is a particularly effective nonverbal gesture to show that you are listening to what the patient is saying and they experience it as a form of recognition. It does not necessarily mean "yes"; it may simply mean "I hear you, please continue." The benefit of head nodding is that without having to say a word, it encourages the patient to continue sharing.

Take Action #1

Head nods coupled with raised eyebrows is a sign of openness and invites a response, or an elaboration on a response.

Today, practice using head nods while your conversational partner is speaking. Keep nodding after the person has finished speaking and remain silent. Note how the individual will likely resume speaking.

6.3.7 Give the Patient Time and Space to Process and Respond

Patients carry a heavy emotional and cognitive load that directly affects their processing time. Mixed emotions, coupled with new vocabulary and novel information, make it difficult for patients to absorb and synthesize information, let alone experience fluency during conversation. For this reason, it is vital to use effective pauses, and even silence at times. Providing patients this gift of time and space during a conversation positively affects their state and enhances processing. It also creates an opening for them to express their needs for information regarding their condition.[6]

Make it a habit to wait a second before commenting or responding to what has been said. This will signal to the patient that you are reflecting on what was shared and that they were heard. It will also prevent you from clipping off the patient's last words, inadvertently communicating that what you had to say was more important. Another advantage of pausing is that it encourages the patient to share more of their concerns, hopes, and values.[7]

Interruption, on the other hand, is a barrier to active listening. Therefore, interrupt only when absolutely necessary because it can be perceived by the patient as dismissive and create an obstacle to connection.

Imagine This #3

Imagine a time when someone has interrupted you while you were experiencing intense feelings or attempting to make an important point. What effect did the interruption have on your state?

6.3.8 Avoid Passing Judgment

In his book, *The Art of Communicating*, Thich Nhat Hanh suggests that when we listen with compassion, our intention must be to help that person suffer less, as well as to avoid getting caught up in judgment.[3] To this end, we must have a sincere desire to understand what the patient is saying while suspending opinions on comments that we find objectionable, offensive, or with which we disagree. Once we form a judgment, everything we hear from that point forward is sifted through our personal filter. We may even begin to search for clues that confirm our judgment and discount any data that oppose it.[8] Left unchecked, our perceptions can perilously distort the patient's reality.

Furthermore, patients have a subconscious awareness of when they are being judged, and thus, they will begin to hold back. Instead, give them the space and freedom to be honest so that you will get a more complete picture of their perspective.

6.3.9 Share the Conversational Floor

When we speak for too long, we unintentionally silence our conversational partner. In the medical setting, information conveyed in a one-way direction toward the patient also places a great deal of strain on listening and subsequently their ability to process and retain information. As a rule, patients can assimilate only two to three critically important pieces of information within a 20-minute period.[6] Research has also suggested that most people can only maintain full attention for three- or four-sentence intervals during a dialogue.[9] After that, attention drops off dramatically. For this reason, limit speaking more than four sentences when a response from the patient has not yet been elicited.

One way to encourage dialogue is to have the patient reflect back their understanding of the information that has been shared. Possible dialogue openers include the following: "I want to be sure I'm explaining things clearly…" or "I've given you a lot of information…."[8] Following this guideline will help improve listening in both you and your patient (▶ Table 6.1).

Take Action #2

Practice the golden rule: Do unto others as you would have others do unto you.

Make a list of all of the compassionate ways you wish people would listen to you (i.e., not interrupting, sharing the conversational floor, asking follow-up questions, showing interest while you speak). Use that same list of skills and practice them on others today. Transfer those same skills to your work with clients.

Table 6.1 Keys to promote attentive listening in patients. Described are communication strategies that support the patient's ability to understand and respond to the health care professional's message

Assess patient's state	Read the patient's nonverbal cues to determine capacity to process information
Consider patient's health literacy	Speak at the patient's language level and use a variety of media
Limit information	Provide only 2–3 important pieces of information over a 20-min period of time
Share the conversational floor	Talk for no more than 2–3 sentences at a time
Request feedback	Engage the patient by soliciting a response: "What are your thoughts…."

6.4 Verbal Behaviors of Active Listening

Feedback is an essential component of good listening. Below are examples of several verbal strategies to use that will signal to the patient that they are seen, heard, and valued, as well as affirm what is being communicated.

6.4.1 Strategies for Verbal Engagement

Providing explanations comprises a large part of a clinician's job. However, the explanations we give are only as productive as the degree to which they provide the patient with the information they want and need to know. The most effective way to find out is to pause our commentary and verbally engage our patients in conversation. Accordingly, Dr. Gurpreet Dhaliwal, a professor of clinical medicine, recommends making a habit of asking these three simple questions (I.C.E.):[10]

• Idea—What is your idea about what is going on?
• Concerns—What are you most worried about?
• Expectations—What are you expecting that I can do?

6.4.2 Reflective Listening Strategies

Reflective listening is critical to instilling a patient's confidence in their caregiver (▶ Fig. 6.1). It can entail simply repeating what the patient says or rephrasing or expanding on the patient's statement.[11] Auguste Fortin VI, MD, professor at the Yale School of Medicine, provides the following example: "...when the patient says, 'Right now, drinking doesn't help me feel better the way it used to. In fact, I feel worse now,' the physician can say, "So drinking is no longer helping you and you want to find some way to feel better instead of drinking."

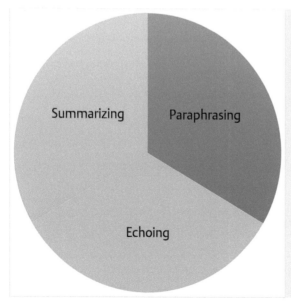

Fig. 6.1 Verbal components of reflective listening. This chart depicts three methods caregivers can use to demonstrate to their patients that they have been heard and understood.

Summarizing

The caregiver ties together the things both the caregiver and the patient have said.[11]

Paraphrasing

This verbal strategy captures the essence of what the patient is saying. It demonstrates what you have gleaned from the patient by repeating back their message in your own words. They will then be able to confirm whether they have been accurately understood.

Echoing

Echoing is considered the shorthand technique of paraphrasing. To echo, you repeat a significant word that the patient has said, like "painful," and then you silently wait for them to further explain the word or subject.

Take Action #3

Practice verbal forms of active listening. Record yourself saying the following words using an upward pitch inflection: Late? Sometimes? Lighter?

Afterward, when you are speaking with a friend and want elaboration on something they just said, repeat the last word your friend said with an upward inflection and pause. Note your friend's response to the technique.

Imagine This #4

Sometimes patients or clients may use their conversational turn to relay a lot of varied information at the same time.

Imagine you are working as a barista and someone steps forward and places this order: "I would like a medium size iced decaf, nonfat soy latte, half sweet with an extra shot, and a caramel drizzle. But please, no foam on top. Oh wait, it doesn't come with foam." What are some of the techniques that could be used to confirm understanding so that the drink is made to the proper specifications?

6.4.3 Acknowledging Statements

These statements can be as simple as, "I hear what you're saying." They do not imply agreement or give judgment of any type, but simply communicate to the patient that they have been heard.

6.4.4 Emotion Labeling

For connection to take place, it is vital to acknowledge the emotions of the patient with whom you are speaking so they feel understood. You can reflect what they are experiencing emotionally by giving their feelings a name, or even better, by labeling the most intense feeling that is being relayed. For example, you might say: "You sound...fearful, concerned, frustrated, angry, or upset...."

Identifying the patient's emotions corroborates what they are feeling instead of minimizing or dismissing it. It also provides an opportunity for the individual to clarify or expound on the feeling.

When you label an emotion, however, be careful to name and identify it with the correct gravitas. If, for example, the patient bellows that they are furious, and then you repeat that they are annoyed, they may feel misunderstood and that their emotions are being downplayed.

6.4.5 Open-Ended and Clarifying Questions

Successful communication takes place only when caregivers accurately understand and incorporate the information gathered from the patient.[12] Asking on-topic questions will demonstrate that you have been paying attention. Additionally, posing open-ended and clarifying questions, like "You mentioned you were feeling..., can you tell me more about that?" signals interest, as well as the desire to accurately and/or fully understand the patient's perspective and what they are communicating.

6.4.6 Minimal Encouragers

These are brief acknowledging comments like "Yes," "Uh-huh," "Oh?" "Really!", and "Wow!" They are not only reassuring to the patient, but also potentially inspire the patient to continue speaking or to open up.

Summary

Active listening is a precious gift to a patient who is experiencing fear, anxiety, frustration, helplessness, or a myriad of other difficult emotions. Attending verbally and nonverbally to the patient attunes the caregiver to the patient's perspective by providing them a safe context to reveal their desires, beliefs, and fears. This in turn encourages the most appropriate response to the patient's needs.

Engaging in careful listening, however, is a conscious, compassionate choice on the part of the caregiver. It is one that promotes connection and trust in the patient who requires healing not just of the body but also of the mind.

References

[1] Doty JR. Into the Magic Shop: A Neurosurgeon's Quest to discover the mysteries of the brain and the secrets of the heart. New York, NY: Avery, an imprint of Penguin Random House; 2017

[2] Nitzky A. The importance of listening in healthcare. http://www.confidentvoices.com/2016/10/30/the-importance-of-listening-in-healthcare/ Published 2016. Accessed July 24, 2017

[3] Hanh N. The art of communicating. New York, NY: HarperCollins; 2014

[4] Covey, S. 7 habits of highly effective people. New York, NY: Simon & Schuster Inc.; 2017

[5] Goman CK. The nonverbal advantage: secrets and science of body language at work. San Francisco, CA: Berrett-Koehler Publishers, Inc.; 2008

[6] Gerteis M, Edgman-Levitan S, Daley J, Delbanco T, eds. Through the patients' eyes: understanding and promoting patient-centered care. San Francisco, CA: Jossey-Bass; 1993

[7] October TW, Dizon ZB, Arnold RM, Rosenberg AR. Characteristics of physician empathetic statements during pediatric intensive care conferences with family members: a qualitative study. JAMA Netw Open. 2018; 1(3): e180351

[8] Boissy A, Gilligan T. Communication the Cleveland clinic way: how to drive a relationship-centered strategy for superior patient experience. New York, NY: McGraw-Hill Education; 2016

[9] Meyers P, Nix S. As we speak: how to make your point and have it stick. New York, NY: Atria Paperback; 2012

[10] The Experts: How to Improve Doctor-Patient Communication. The Wall Street Journal. https://www.wsj.com/articles/SB10001424127887324050304578411251805908228 Published 2013. Accessed January 6, 2016

[11] Tucker ME. Motivational interviewing promotes patient behavior change. https://www.medscape.com/viewarticle/863064. Published 2016. Accessed February 9, 2017

[12] The Joint Commission. Advancing effective communication, cultural competence, and patient- and family-centered care: A roadmap for hospitals. Oakbrook Terrace, IL: The Joint Commission; 2010

Chapter 7

Using Vocal Tone that Reflects Empathy

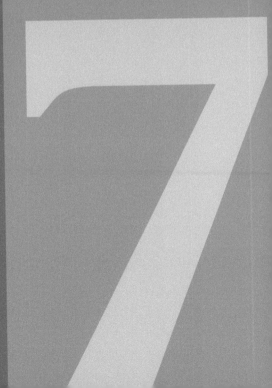

7 Using Vocal Tone that Reflects Empathy

Abstract
This chapter explores the nonlinguistic signals of voice—style and tone—and their critical role in communicating with compassion. Speaking with an empathetic vocal tone can provide the much-needed comfort and consolation required for the patients' healing process. Adjustments can also be made to speaking style. This chapter describes how altering the pacing and pausing of speech can improve both the clarity of a message and the patient's processing of information during patient–provider communication. This chapter also explores the significant effects of intention and emotion on vocal tone—two elements that cause the voice to change involuntarily. Caregivers must therefore be aware of their state as they enter into patient interactions, knowing that how they feel inwardly will naturally be reflected in the tone of voice they use with the patient. Patients, in turn, will form an opinion of their caregiver based on their perception of the caregiver's voice and whether it reflects the necessary authentic care and concern that engenders trust and respect.

Keywords: nonlinguistic signals of voice, tone of voice, vocal tone, communicating with compassion, empathetic vocal tone, patient–provider communication, healing process

It's not what you say, it's how you say it.

Proverb

7.1 Natalie's Story

It was a dreary Monday morning when the lactation consultant dropped in to speak with me. My newborn son and I were set to go home that day, and I was lying still in bed, trying not to trigger any pain from the C-section I had had just a couple of days earlier.

After a curt "good morning," the lactation consultant seated herself clear across the room and asked me how the nursing was going. Well, I knew it wasn't going well at all. The night before, the nurse had brought my son to me several times as I tried to breast-feed him, but he was unable to take anything in. I was deeply frustrated and distressed because I knew he was hungry, and I couldn't provide him with the food he needed. So how did I respond to the consultant's question? I squarely lied and told her everything was going okay. After an uncomfortable pause, she looked me in the eyes, and in a chilling tone I will never forget, she pronounced, "It can't be going that well; your son has lost almost a pound since birth." My heart just sank.

When I think about it now, I realize that my pride had gotten in the way of owning the truth. I was embarrassed for failing at a task I erroneously thought came naturally to new mothers. Did I need the lactation consultant to be truthful with me? Absolutely—but not with that condescending voice or the shaming way she went about it.

A few days following the hospital stay, a home health nurse came to check up on the two of us. I was still so worried about my son's weight, and in my hormonally imbalanced state, questioning whether I was fit to be a mom. The nurse turned out to be more like an angel sent to me in my moment of need. I will forever be grateful that she could sense my struggle and respond to me with a kind, maternal reassurance. I remember before parting, she leaned in toward me and in the most calming and comforting of tones said, "You're both doing just fine."—and that sentiment rang true from that day onward.

7.2 About the Voice

In *The Patient Experience*, author Brian Boyle describes the pivotal role of his caregiver's vocal tone while he was in a medically induced coma.[1] He recounts: "Whoever came into my room, I was instantly attuned to their presence, mood, actions, and especially, their voice... I could immediately tell if they were having a good day or a really bad day, which was reflected in the treatment I received."

Research, in fact, has demonstrated that when compared to communication across multiple senses, perceivers of voice-only communication are the most accurate in detecting other's emotions and intentions.[2] This is attributed to their focus of attention on the one channel of communication. It is also a testament to the abundance of information contained within the human voice.

7.3 The Nonlinguistic Signals of Voice

The nonlinguistic signals of voice—style and tone—highly influence social interactions. Style consists of the pacing and pausing we use, while tone relates to the pitch, loudness, timbre (quality), and resonance. Each signal conveys meaning and emotion. In the health care setting, the sound of our voices can be used as instruments of healing, or sadly, of injury (▶ Fig. 7.1). See ▶ Video 1.2.

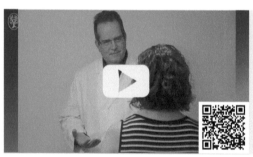

Video 1.2 Using an Empathic Vocal Tone with Patients and video URL: https://www.thieme.de/de/q.htm?p=opn/cs/19/11/10686241-1a15d63f

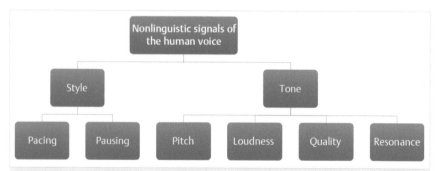

Fig. 7.1 Nonlinguistic signals of the human voice. Listed are the subcomponents of vocal style and tone.

Tonal qualities of concern/anxiety are believed to be positively related to feelings of empathy, whereas deep, loud, and moderately fast speech are associated with dominance and lack of empathy. The patient's perception of the caregiver's voice directly influences their feelings toward the caregiver. In fact, one study revealed the provider's harsh tone, more than the content of the conversation, to be a predictor of malpractice claims.[3] This is a clear illustration of how the tone of voice a caregiver uses when communicating with patients is as important as the information they are conveying.

7.3.1 Relationship between Vocal Tone and Emotion

Also referred to as emotional prosody, our tone of voice reflects what we are feeling on the inside (▶ Fig. 7.2). Across cultures, there exists a universality in the voice production (pitch, loudness, and speech rate) for the basic emotions of fear, anger, happiness, and sadness.[4] Just as the lips, the eyes, the eyebrows, etc., create a visual display of our emotions, vocal cues perform the same function auditorily. The area in our brain stem that is responsible for the autonomic fight or flight response is the same area where the nuclei for tone of voice and facial expression reside.[5] Consequently, when we experience an emotion, both change without our conscious effort.

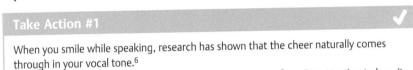

Take Action #1 ✔

When you smile while speaking, research has shown that the cheer naturally comes through in your vocal tone.[6]

The next time you pick up the phone, put a smile on your face. Pay attention to how it brightens your tone. Also, request a friend to call you twice. During the first call, say the sentence, "Hello... how is your day going?" while smiling. During the next call, say the same sentence without smiling. Could your friend detect the difference in your vocal tone?

Our vocal tone will not hide our emotions—it will display them. For instance, when we are clutched by a feeling, physiological changes in heart rate, blood flow, and muscle tension occur that alter the shape, functionality, and sound of the vocal mechanism.[7] All arise without our immediate awareness or choice. Evidence of this includes when

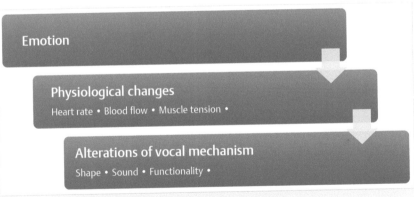

Fig. 7.2 Effects of emotion on vocal tone. Illustrated are the bodily reactions to emotion that impact the vocal mechanism and result in variations of vocal tone.

you may have inadvertently spoken in a loud voice when excited or talked with an uncharacteristically high-pitched voice when feeling intimidated, or perhaps spoken with vocal tremor during a presentation.

7.3.2 Vocal Perception

Like facial expression, patients make snap judgments about the caregiver's personality based on vocal tone. In fact, judgments can be made in less than a second of hearing an individual's voice.[8] Literally, within the time it takes an individual to say "hello," they will subconsciously make judgments about traits like aggression and trustworthiness.[9]

Discrimination among vocal expressions begins as early as infancy.[10] The amygdala and auditory areas of the brain code the emotion-related acoustic information such as fluctuations in voice quality (i.e., shrill, harsh, or soft), loudness, and pitch.[11] These tonal variations are perceived during speech, as well as during nonword utterances called vocal bursts—involuntary sounds like shrieks, groans, grunts, or the breathy "whaaaaa."[12]

Outcomes from perceptual tests reveal that listeners can quickly and easily assess a person's emotional state based on these subtleties of vocal tone.[13] An example of this is when we are able to discern a loved one's mood simply by their tone when answering the phone.

Imagine This #1

Imagine a time you called a loved one on the phone and you knew immediately something was wrong when you heard the individual say "hello."

Another perfect illustration of our ability to pick up on subtle nuances of emotional prosody is when we sense emptiness behind the words being spoken. The receiver may hear one thing, but the heart feels something totally different. This occurs when the words an individual says and the vocal tone and style used to deliver the words impart contradictory messages. One clear illustration is when you may have been greeted with, "Good morning," only to walk away certain it was not a good morning at all for that person. Undoubtedly you subconsciously picked up on nonverbal signals of vocal tone (and possibly facial expression) that did not align with the individual's verbal expression.

7.3.3 Using the Voice Mindfully

It is imperative to have a level of self-awareness relative to personal mindset and emotional state as we enter different patient situations, because both can easily be detected in our voices. When there is empathy in our hearts, the compassion echoes in our vocal tone. Conversely, a negative tone resonates when we harbor adverse emotions such as impatience, annoyance, and judgment.

7.3.4 Intention and Vocal Tone

As caregivers, we use a lot of scripted phrases throughout the day, and when they are not infused with kindness and compassion, they can be perceived as sterile. Patients instantly know whether we truly care when we ask, "How are you feeling today?" because it is very difficult to simulate the sound of an emotion if it is contrary to how we are feeling.[14] As a rule, only trained actors are able to accomplish this, and only by recalling a past event in their life.[14]

How can we make our voices sound more empathic and caring? One of the most effective ways to soften our voices is by considering the patient's perspective or imagining how we would feel if the patient in front of us was a loved one.

Take Action #2

Imagine yourself in the presence of a loved one who is vulnerable due to age or physical state. Then record yourself saying the following statements and questions using an empathetic tone of voice:

- How can I help you?
- How are you feeling today?
- Where are you hurting?
- Let's try it this way.
- Let me repeat that for you.

By envisioning your loved one, were you able to achieve the gentle vocal affect you desired?

7.3.5 Monitoring Speech Rate

Due to body–mind feedback, vocal expansiveness, such as speaking slowly and using pauses, has been found to positively affect the way we think, feel, and behave. At the same time, researchers have found that this type of speech reflects an openness to others, and even a willingness to be interrupted.[15] Furthermore, in the medical setting, it significantly improves the patient's ability to hear more clearly and to understand forthcoming information. For this reason, make it a point to never speak at a faster rate than the patient. Studies show that others also feel "pressured" when someone speaks more quickly than they do.[16]

Imagine This #2

Imagine being in the process of an important transaction that affects you personally, but of which you have rudimentary knowledge and experience, that is, speaking with a financial advisor, leasing a car, or purchasing a computer or an internet package. What kind of vocal tone and style would you like the individual with whom you are interacting to use? Consider this when you are explaining critical information to your client or patient.

7.3.6 Mirroring Vocal Style and Tone

Social scientists regard mimicry as a natural act that engenders trust. Intonation, voice inflection, speed of speaking, and even accents can all be synchronized.

When it comes to building rapport with others, mirroring these vocal elements has been shown to be as effective as mirroring body language. Studies performed in a variety of service industries have demonstrated the positive effects of the mirroring process on connecting with others. For example, both waitstaff and salespeople who mimic the verbal style of their customers reap the rewards in extra tips and sales, respectively.[17] In the health care setting, synching our vocal patterns to our patients has been proven beneficial to communication as it promotes both understanding and being understood.

7.3.7 Using Pauses for Emphasis

One way to modify speech rate is through pausing. Used strategically, it can improve the clarity of a message. Pauses alert the patient that what you are about to say is important and naturally break messages into short statements that are more easily assimilated.

Summary

The expression and perception of emotional states when we speak are fundamental aspects of patient–caregiver communication. A pleasant vocal tone can provide comfort and consolation to patients and plays a notable role in the patient's recovery process. In addition, adjustments such as pauses, and providing explanations at a slower speaking rate, can be used to improve the overall quality of the communication.

References

[1] Boyle B. The patient experience: the importance of care, communication, and compassion in the hospital room. New York, NY: Skyhorse Publishing; 2015

[2] Kraus MW. Voice-only communication enhances empathic accuracy. Am Psychol. 2017; 72(7):644–654

[3] Ambady N, Laplante D, Nguyen T, Rosenthal R, Chaumeton N, Levinson W. Surgeons' tone of voice: a clue to malpractice history. Surgery. 2002; 132(1):5–9

[4] Matsumoto D, Frank MG, Hwang HS. Nonverbal communication: science and applications. Los Angeles, CA: Sage; 2013

[5] Riess H. The power of empathy: Helen Riess at TEDxMiddlebury [video]. Youtube. https://www.youtube.com/watch?v=baHrcC8B4WM Published December 12, 2013. Accessed March 18, 2018

[6] Drahota A, Costall A, Reddy V. The vocal communication of different kinds of smile. Speech Commun. 2008; 50(4):278–287

[7] Schirmer A, Kotz SA. Beyond the right hemisphere: brain mechanisms mediating vocal emotional processing. Trends Cogn Sci. 2006; 10(1):24–30

[8] Thomson H. Your voice betrays your personality in a split second. https://www.newscientist.com/article/dn25226-your-voice-betrays-your-personality-in-a-split-second/. Published 2014. Accessed November 6, 2016

[9] Trudeau M. You had me at hello: the science behind first impressions. http://www.npr.org/sections/health-shots/2014/05/05/308349318/you-had-me-at-hello-the-science-behind-first-impressions. Published 2014. Accessed May 21, 2016

[10] Grossmann T. The development of emotion perception in face and voice during infancy. Restor Neurol Neurosci. 2010; 28(2):219–236

[11] Bestelmeyer PE, Maurage P, Rouger J, Latinus M, Belin P. Adaptation to vocal expressions reveals multistep perception of auditory emotion. J Neurosci. 2014; 34(24):8098–8105

[12] Simon-Thomas ER, Keltner DJ, Sauter D, Sinicropi-Yao L, Abramson A. The voice conveys specific emotions: evidence from vocal burst displays. Emotion. 2009; 9(6):838–846

[13] Bachorowski J. Vocal expression and perception of emotion. Curr Dir Psychol Sci. 1999; 8(2):53–57

[14] Ekman P. Emotions revealed: recognizing faces and feelings to improve communication and emotional life. New York, NY: St. Martin's Griffin; 2007

[15] Guillory LE, Gruenfeld DH. Fake it till you make it: how acting powerful leads to feeling empowered [manuscript]. Stanford, CA: Stanford Graduate School of Business, Stanford; 2010

[16] Pease A, Pease B. The definitive book of body language. New York, NY: Bantam Books; 2006

[17] Cialdini RB. Pre-suasion: A revolutionary way to influence and persuade. New York, NY: Simon & Schuster Paperbacks; 2018

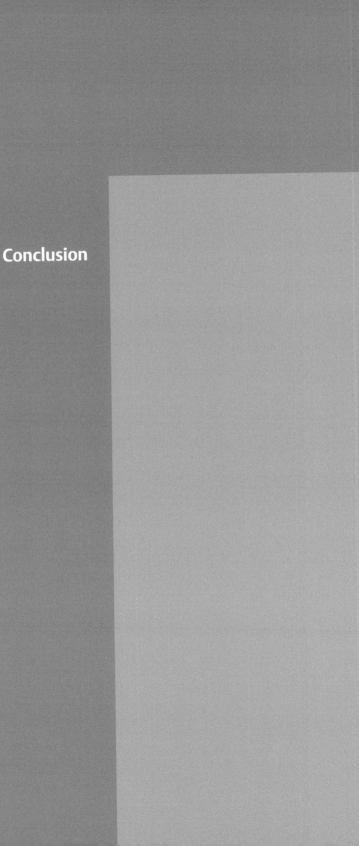

Conclusion

Conclusion

Every act of compassion, every intention to serve, is a gift to this world and a gift to yourself.

James Doty, MD

Caregivers can be true agents of healing when they possess a firm desire and commitment to be of service and to ease the suffering of those entrusted in their care. Engaging in this compassionate care, however, calls upon a myriad of efficacious verbal and non-verbal communication skills. The ability to listen with empathy, and to express kindness and warmth through eye contact, facial expression, vocal tone and touch, for example, helps provide much needed comfort and consolation. Together, these communicative acts engender trust that leads to bonding between the patient and the caregiver.

Furthermore, communication that reflects a caring attitude helps heal more than just the ailing body. It treats patients as "whole" individuals, addressing not only their physical concerns but also their social and emotional needs. By demonstrating attitudes and behaviors that are sensitive to their values, customs, and ethnic backgrounds, caregivers can help their patients feel understood and supported. Considering the patient's perspective of their illness is also an integral component to the healing process. For instance, the acceptance and compliance of the treatment plan greatly improves when the caregiver considers the patient's beliefs surrounding their illness and therapeutic preferences.

Compassionate communication is a win–win proposition; in addition to fueling the body, soul, and spirit of the patient, it positively influences the caregivers' well-being. By empathically participating in the therapeutic process, we experience physiological gains as well as the intrinsic rewards of being open, kind, and fully present. Through the seven keys of compassionate communication, caregivers deepen their connection with patients—ultimately bringing meaning and purpose to our work and to our lives.

Index

Note: Page numbers set **bold** or *italic* indicate headings or figures, respectively.